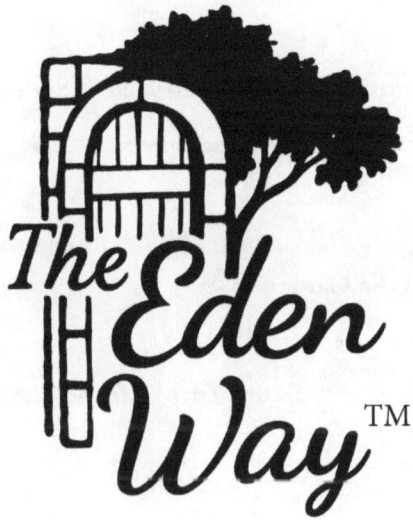

The Eden Way™

Other Works by Angel Tate Keaton

Resources to help you return to the Creator's original design for body, mind, and spirit.

The Eden Way™ Series

Book 1-*The Eden Way™: Reclaiming Body, Mind, and Spirit Through the Creator's Original Design*

Book 2-*The Eden Way™ Journal: 49-Days to Reset Body, Mind, and Spirit* (Companion to Book 1)

RISE: Rooted, Intentional, Strong, Energized™ Series

Book 1-*RISE™ Wellness Journal — Rooted, Intentional, Strong, Energized™: Embrace One Year of Habits, Healing, and Hope*

The Little Keepers of the Garden™

Book 1-*The Little Keepers of the Garden™: Seeds of Truth Collection*

The Little Keepers of the Garden™: Seeds of Truth Collection Activity Book (Companion to Book 1)

Explore all titles and resources at HealthyInHeart.com

Thank you for beginning the journey with me. Your heart matters. Your healing matters. Let's walk Eden's path together.

THE EDEN WAY
Reclaiming Body, Mind, and Spirit

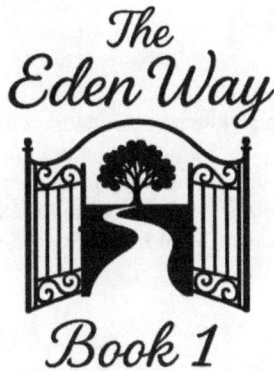

The
Eden Way

Book 1

Through the Creator's Original Design

~

ANGEL TATE KEATON

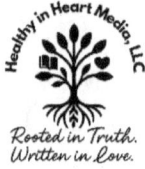

Published in the United States of America by
Healthy in Heart Media
P.O. Box 694
Vinton, VA 24179
Copyright © 2025 by Angel Tate Keaton
First Printing, September 2025
Cover art and design by the author

Rooted in Truth.
Written in Love.

Library of Congress Control Number: 2025915919

ISBN— 978-1-969064-00-5

Disclaimer

The author of this book does not dispense medical advice or prescribe the use of any technique as a form of treatment for medical, emotional, psychological, or physical conditions without the guidance of a licensed physician or qualified healthcare provider, either directly or indirectly. The intent of the author is solely to offer information of a general nature to support you in your personal journey toward emotional, physical, mental, and spiritual well-being.

If you choose to apply any of the information presented in this book, you do so of your own volition. The author and the publisher assume no responsibility for your actions or any consequences that may arise from the use or misuse of the information contained herein.

Scripture Notice

Unless otherwise noted, all Scripture quotations are taken from the American Standard Version (ASV), as provided by BibleGateway.com. The American Standard Version was originally published in 1901 and is now in the public domain. This version was chosen for its consistent use of the divine name in the Old Testament and its closer alignment with the original Hebrew, making it a suitable foundation for a return-to-Eden perspective.

DEDICATION

To my beloved husband,

Todd

Thank you for walking this journey beside me—

in the garden seasons and the wilderness ones.

Your support, encouragement, and steady faith

have been a covering of peace in every step of this calling.

Thank you for making space

in our home, in your heart, and in your schedule,

enabling me to pour out these words.

You have not only supported my writing,

you have lived it with me.

This book is ours.

With deepest love, honor, and gratitude,

Angel

**To our daughter,
Kelsey**

Your light, laughter, and fierce spirit
have been a constant joy on this journey.

Thank you for inspiring me to live what I write,
and for reminding me why truth matters.

You are one of my greatest gifts
and one of my clearest reasons to keep going.

With all my love,
Mom

ACKNOWLEDGMENTS

First and foremost, I give thanks to YHVH, the Creator of heaven and earth, who opened my eyes to see, my ears to hear, and my heart to receive. It is by His Spirit that I have been given the sight to perceive His messages and the wisdom to discern the Truth. Without Him, these words would be empty.

To my parents, Ray (of blessed memory) and Rachel—thank you for planting the seeds of faith early in my life, for teaching me that not only does our Creator exist, but that I could know Him personally. That foundation became the soil where deeper roots of truth and understanding could grow.

To Ross K. Nichols, Dr. James D. Tabor, and all the teachers whose wisdom has guided me, near and far, I offer my heartfelt gratitude. Your words, your questions, and your faithfulness have helped shape my own. And to those whose views have challenged mine—thank you. You pushed me to search harder, dig deeper, and hold fast only to what is true.

To the Yachad, whose encouragement gave wind to these pages—you reminded me that passion is worth putting into words, and that purpose is worth pursuing.

With a heart full of gratitude, I offer this work not as a final word, but as one voice among many—yearning, seeking, learning, and longing to walk in Truth.

Contents

OTHER WORKS BY ANGEL TATE KEATON II

INTRODUCTION 1

WHY NOT YOU? WHY NOT NOW? 1

1—BACK TO THE BEGINNING: WHY EDEN STILL MATTERS 6

I.   THE BLUEPRINT OF EDEN 6
      The Original Health Plan 6
      Whole, Unashamed, Nourished, Connected 7
      What Does "Very Good" Actually Mean? 8
II.   FOUR CORNERSTONES OF EDENIC HEALTH 9
      1.   Plant-Based Nourishment 9
      2.   Purposeful Movement and Stewardship 10
      3.   Emotional Integrity (No Shame, Fear, or Blame) 11
      4.   Spiritual Intimacy (Daily Communion with YHVH) 11
III. WHY WE LONG FOR EDEN 12
      The Ache of Disconnection 13
      Eternity Set in Our Hearts 14
      Modern Symptoms of Eden Lost 14
IV.   THE GOOD NEWS: EDEN ISN'T GONE... IT'S CALLING 15
      Yeshua and the Tree of Life: A Living Teaching 15

2—THE FALL: ROOT OF DISEASE, DISTORTION, AND DISCONNECT 19

I. WHAT REALLY BROKE IN THE GARDEN 19
      The Turning Point: "Did Elohim Really Say...?" 19
      What Was Lost in One Moment 20
      The High Cost of Disobedience 22
      But the Story Didn't End There 23
II. THE THREEFOLD DEATH 23
      This is the Threefold Death: physical, emotional, and spiritual 24
      Why the Threefold Death Matters 27
III. GENERATIONAL PATTERNS AND MODERN MANIFESTATIONS 27
      The Torah Shows the Pattern of Inheritance 28
      Breaking the Pattern 31
IV. HOPE FORESHADOWED 31
      Garments of Grace 32
      The Promise of Restoration 32

Messiah: The One Who Laid Down His Life to End Death's Reign..................33

The Garden Was Closed—But the Way Was Not Lost.....................34

3—THE GARDEN DIET: WHY FOOD IS SPIRITUAL **35**

I. FOOD AS DIVINE ASSIGNMENT 35

Food as a Sacred Starting Point...35

The Edenic Diet: Plant-Based and Blood-Free.............................36

Eating as Worship and Obedience..37

The Daily Choice to Align or Depart..37

II. THE SPIRITUAL WEIGHT OF EATING 38

Leviticus Food Laws: Discernment, Holiness, and Vitality 38

Acts 15: Food and the Gentile Believers 39

Why YHVH Cares What We Eat..40

Eating as a Form of Worship..41

III. BLOOD, LIFE, AND THE HEART OF THE FATHER...........................41

The Body Is Bathed in Blood—Every Cell, Every Fiber..................42

The Prohibition of Blood Consumption 42

Animal Death Post-Fall: A Mercy and a Consequence...................43

Yeshua's Teachings on the Restoration of Life............................44

The Heart of the Father Has Always Been Life 45

IV. EATING AS ALIGNMENT 45

Eating as a Spiritual Act of Alignment 46

Healing the Gut—and the Soul—With Edenic Food.......................47

The Daily Return 47

4—THE SILENT SABOTEURS: HIDDEN POISONS IN MODERN FOOD....................**49**

I. THE CHEMISTRY OF COMPROMISE..49

II. SPIRITUAL CONSEQUENCES OF EATING WHAT WAS NEVER FOOD.............50

III. FROM SLAVERY TO STEWARDSHIP 50

V.   CREATING A DETOX PLAN..50

Pantry Purge 51

Budget Meal Prep..51

Gentle Healing Tools..51

Rebuild with Real Food 51

VI. WHEN THE VESSEL POISONS THE OFFERING: TOXINS IN COOKWARE AND STORAGE 52

Plastic Storage Containers and Utensils 52

Aluminum Cookware 52

Copper Cookware 52

SAFER ALTERNATIVES 53

5—UNDOING BABYLON: ESCAPING THE LIES OF MODERN WELLNESS............. 54

I. RECOGNIZING BABYLON'S INFLUENCE 54

Confusion: The Signature of Babylon 55

Excess: When "More" Becomes the Disease 55

Performance: The Disguised Idol of Modern Health 56

Pharmakeia: The False Priesthood of Healing 56

II. DIET CULTURE VS. EDENIC CULTURE 58

Shame-Based Restrictions vs. Creator-Based Nourishment 58

Idolatry of Body Image, Industry, and "Self-Care"....................... 59

Eden Invites, Diet Culture Demands 60

III. DETOXING THE BODY AND THE BELIEFS 61

Processed Food and Pharmaceutical Dependency......................... 61

Spiritual Detox: Repentance, Renewal, Reorientation 63

This Is Not About Perfection. It's About Realignment 64

IV. RETURNING TO SIMPLICITY AND TRUTH.. 64

Daniel's Diet as Resistance 65

Real Food, Real Faith, Real Freedom.. 66

Eden Isn't Complicated. Babylon Is 67

V. PROCEED WITH WISDOM: A NOTE ON MEDICATION AND HEALING 68

6—THE MIND OF MESSIAH: BREAKING MENTAL STRONGHOLDS..................... 71

I. RENEWAL AS TRANSFORMATION 71

What Is a Stronghold?... 72

The Mind of Messiah: What It Means to Renew 72

The Difference Between Thoughts and Truth 73

Transformation Begins in the Mind 74

II. EMOTIONAL SABOTAGE PATTERNS.. 75

Negative Self-Talk: The Inner Critic Masquerading as Truth 76

Shame Cycles: The Lie That You Are Your Mistakes 77

Anxiety Loops: The Mind Racing on a Treadmill of Fear 77

Root Causes: Trauma, Lies, and Spiritual Influence 78

Healing Begins with Awareness... 79

III. YESHUA'S MINDSET 80

Humility: Letting Go of the Need to Prove.................................. 81

Surrender: Aligning With the Father's Will.................................. 82

Peace: A Settled Mind in an Unsettled World.............................. 82

Alignment With Truth and Purpose 83

IV. WARFARE AND IDENTITY 84

Spiritual Battle in the Tanakh.. 85

Replacing Lies with Truth-Based Declarations 85

Journaling Stronghold Breakthroughs 86

You Are Not a Victim in This Battle 88

7—THE EMOTIONAL BODY: WHEN FEELINGS BECOME PHYSICAL 89

I. THE PSYCHOSOMATIC CONNECTION 89

Stress, Trauma, and Chronic Inflammation 90

Nervous System Responses and Cellular Memory 90

The Body Doesn't Lie—It Speaks 92

II. CASE STUDIES: WHEN THE BODY SPEAKS 92

Eczema and Emotional Triggers 93

Autoimmunity and Self-Rejection 93

Gut Health and Unprocessed Grief 94

Anne's Story: Hashimoto's Thyroiditis and the Edenic Diet 95

The Body as Prophet, Not Enemy 96

III. INNER HEALING FOR OUTER RESTORATION 97

Forgiveness: Releasing What Was Never Yours to Carry 97

Repentance: Returning to Truth and Alignment 98

Grief Work: Making Space for What Was Lost 99

Psalm 139: YHVH Knows Every Part 99

IV. TOOLS FOR HEALING THE EMOTIONAL BODY 100

Breathwork: Resetting the Nervous System 100

Journaling: Releasing What the Body Carries 101

Safe Boundaries: Honoring the Body's Yes and No 102

Emotions as Messengers, Not Enemies 103

8—THE SABBATH RHYTHM OF HEALING 104

I. THE PATTERN FROM THE BEGINNING 104

Rest as a Sacred Rhythm 105

Exodus 20: Sabbath as Commandment and Gift 105

II. THE HEALING SCIENCE OF REST 106

Hormonal Reset: Cortisol, Insulin, and Sleep 106

Nervous System Regulation and Trauma Healing 107

Rest as Recovery, Not Reward 108

III. RHYTHMS OF SURRENDER 108

Letting Go of Control 109

Receiving Joy 109

Stillness as Strength 110

Trust: The Foundation of Sabbath 110

IV. MAKING SABBATH HOLY AGAIN... 111

    Sabbath Preparation: Rest Begins Before Sundown 111

    Sabbath Foods: Nourishment Without Stress..................... 112

    Rituals That Set the Day Apart....................................... 112

    Heart Postures: Resting in Trust..................................... 113

9—LIVING WATER & LIVING WORDS 115

I. WATER AS A PHYSICAL AND SPIRITUAL SYMBOL 115

    Water at the Beginning 115

    Water in the Womb... 116

    Mikveh: Immersion and Renewal................................... 116

    Yeshua and Living Water 117

    Hydration and Cellular Healing..................................... 117

    Restoring the Waters Within 118

II. THE POWER OF SPEECH... 118

    Self-Talk: When You Preach to Yourself 119

    Prayer: Language of Intimacy and Authority..................... 120

    Declarations: Speaking Life on Purpose 120

    Your Voice Restores Atmospheres.................................. 121

III. YHVH'S NAME AND HEALING AUTHORITY 122

    The Tetragrammaton: Breath, Being, and Frequency........... 122

    Titles vs. the True Name 123

    Healing and the Name.. 123

    Speaking the Name with Reverence and Boldness 124

IV. WORDS THAT HEAL 124

    Blessing the Body 125

    Speaking Truth to Trauma 125

    The Word Made Flesh 126

10—FROM SURVIVING TO SOVEREIGNTY 128

I. THE SHIFT FROM VICTIM TO STEWARD................................. 128

    From Survival Mode to Kingdom Mode........................... 129

    Taking Dominion Starts with You.................................. 129

    Breaking Passive Patterns 130

II. SOVEREIGNTY OVER THE FLESH 131

    Choosing Obedience Over Craving 131

    Training the Body... 132

    Renewing Discipline Through Delight 133

    From Flesh-Driven to Spirit-Led.................................... 133

III. SOVEREIGNTY OVER THE MIND AND EMOTIONS 133

    Emotions as Tools, Not Tyrants.. 134

    Setting Boundaries: Guarding the Garden Within 135

    Affirming Identity: Knowing Who You Are................................ 135

    From Turmoil to Shalom 136

IV. AUTHORITY IN THE SPIRIT 136

    Prayers of Binding and Loosing.. 137

    Spiritual Gifts in Healing and Restoration............................ 137

    Walking in Spiritual Dominion... 138

11—MAKING YOUR HOME EDEN AGAIN **140**

I. YOUR ENVIRONMENT MATTERS 140

    The Space Around You Reflects the Space Within........................ 140

    Healing Requires a Safe Nest 141

    Peace, Order, and Purity: The Edenic Blueprint 141

    Making Eden Tangible 142

II. DETOXING THE HOME 143

    The Hidden Toxins in Your Home.. 143

    Creating a Low-Inflammation Kitchen................................... 145

    Detoxing the Bathroom and Laundry Space 146

    Making the Shift Sustainable 146

SECTION III 147

    What Makes a Space Sacred?.. 147

    The Sensory Anchors of Sanctuary 148

    Rhythms that Invite Shalom.. 148

    How a Sanctuary Heals... 149

    Restoring Eden Room by Room 150

IV. CREATING A SAFE PLACE FOR THE SOUL.................................. 150

    Hospitality to the Ruach (Holy Spirit) 150

    Sanctuary Over Showcase... 151

    Creating That Safe Place.. 152

12—COMMUNITY: HEALING BEYOND THE SELF **153**

I. THE ORIGINAL DESIGN: MADE FOR RELATIONSHIP 153

    Eden Was a Fellowship 154

    The Wound of Isolation.. 154

    The Circle Restored 155

    From Me to We 155

II. THE WOUNDS OF DISCONNECTION 156

Loneliness as an Inflammatory, Emotional Burden *156*

The Cost of Broken Trust *158*

From Walls to Bridges *158*

You Were Never Meant to Heal Alone *159*

III. BUILDING AN EDENIC CIRCLE *159*

Spiritual Friendships vs. Codependent Entanglements *159*

What a Safe Community Looks Like *160*

Spiritual Friendship vs. Codependent Entanglement *160*

Sharing Meals, Worship, and Rest in Rhythm *161*

Rebuilding Eden Together *162*

IV. ACCOUNTABILITY AND INTERCESSION *162*

Confess, Pray, and Stand Together *163*

Spiritual Warfare Isn't Meant to Be Solo *163*

Vulnerable and Powerful — At the Same Time *164*

The Commission of Community *164*

V. CREATING SPACES OF HEALING FOR OTHERS *165*

Being Willing to Be Seen, Known, and Sent *165*

Your Healing Is Someone Else's Breakthrough *166*

Restoration as Reproduction *166*

Be Seen, Be Known, Be Sent *167*

This Is How the Garden Grows *167*

13—CREATION HEALS: RETURNING TO THE NATURAL WORLD **169**

I. THE PHYSIOLOGY OF RECONNECTION *170*

Forest Bathing and Nervous System Calm *170*

Grounding and Cellular Balance *170*

Circadian Rhythms and Sunlight *170*

The Power of Fresh Air *171*

II. GARDENING: THERAPY AND SPIRITUAL DISCIPLINE *171*

III. NATURE REFLECTS THE VOICE OF THE CREATOR *171*

IV. RETURNING TO EDEN THROUGH CREATION *172*

V. THE GARDEN WAS ALWAYS PART OF THE PLAN *173*

VI. CREATION AND EMOTIONAL REGULATION *173*

Beauty as Emotional Medicine *173*

Stillness for Inner Stability *173*

Nature as Safe Attachment *174*

VII. DIGITAL OVERLOAD VS. DIVINE DESIGN *174*

The Opposite of Eden *175*

Micro-Sabbaths in Nature *175*

Neuroplasticity Through Nature *175*

VIII. CHILDREN AND CREATION: RESTORING WONDER EARLY 175

    Developmental Need, Not Luxury *176*

    Teach Through Tending *176*

IX. CREATION AND WORSHIP: REKINDLING AWE 176

X. REWILDING THE SOUL 177

14—PLANTING EDEN IN THE NEXT GENERATION **178**

I. A HOME THAT FEELS LIKE EDEN 179

II. PROTECTING DEVELOPING MINDS 180

III. TEACHING RHYTHMS OF EDEN EARLY 181

IV. HEALING THE PARENT TO RAISE THE CHILD 182

THE GARDEN IS MEANT TO GROW 183

SABBATH ACTIVITY GUIDE FOR KIDS 183

    Friday Night Prep (Erev Shabbat) *184*

    Shabbat Morning *184*

    Creative Quiet Time *184*

    Afternoon Peace Activities *185*

    Suggested Sabbath Read-Aloud Books *185*

OPTIONAL PREPARATION TOOLS FOR PARENTS 186

15—GRIEVING WHAT WAS LOST: WHEN HEALING INCLUDES LAMENT **187**

I. GRIEVING THE BODY YOU ABUSED OR NEGLECTED 188

II. GRIEVING BETRAYAL, CHURCH WOUNDS, AND CHILDHOOD TRAUMA 188

III. THE ROLE OF TEARS IN DETOX AND HEALING 189

IV. SCRIPTURAL LAMENTS: MODELS FOR EMOTIONAL RELEASE 190

V. A SAFE PLACE TO WEEP 190

VI.   THE GARDEN INCLUDED SORROW 191

    How to Write a Psalm of Lament *191*

    Writing Prompts *192*

16—THE EDEN TO COME: LONGING FOR THE FINAL GARDEN **194**

I.   THE TREE OF LIFE REAPPEARS 194

II.   WHY OUR SMALL STEPS STILL MATTER 195

III. THE TENSION OF "NOW AND NOT YET" 196

IV. LIVING PROPHETICALLY: EDEN NOW 197

V. THE TABLE OF THE KINGDOM 198

VI. WHY NOT NOW? WHY NOT HERE? 199

17—WHEN EDEN FEELS FAR: STAYING FAITHFUL IN THE STRUGGLE **200**

I. Healing Isn't Linear 201

II. When Others Don't Come with You... 202

III. The Trap of Perfectionism 203

IV. How to Show Up When It's Hard 203

V. Rebuilding Trust: With YHVH and Your Body.............................. 205

    Final Encouragement... 206

18—STEWARDING EDEN: TIME, MONEY, AND THE WEIGHT OF ENOUGH 208

I. Budgeting for Wellness: Eden on a Modest Income....................... 209

II. Sabbath: Resetting Time and Breaking Work Addiction 210

III. Escaping Consumerism in the Wellness World 211

IV. Making Peace with Small Beginnings.. 212

V. Trading Scarcity for Trust 213

    Practical Stewardship Reflections 214

    Final Encouragement... 215

19—WALKING IT OUT: TESTIMONIES, TOOLS, AND TRANSFORMATION........... 216

I. Real Stories of Edenic Renewal 216

    My Story: From Breakdown to Blueprint.. 217

    Testimony from My Husband, Todd.. 217

    Others Who Reclaimed Wholeness 218

II. Practical Tools and Templates.. 221

    1. Daily Rhythm Guides 222

    2. Edenic Recipes and Pantry Lists 223

    3. Spiritual Declarations 224

    4. Prayer Templates 225

III. Journal Prompts and Action Plans... 226

    Why Journaling Matters on This Journey 226

    Action Planning: From Insight to Implementation 228

    Encouragement for the Hard Days... 229

IV. Commissioning and Invitation... 230

    A Call to Keep Walking 230

    Eden Was Never Meant to Stay Lost... 231

    An Invitation Forward 231

20—WHY NOT HERE? WHY NOT NOW? 233

The Prophets' Vision of Eden and the Call to Us Today 233

I. The Prophets' Vision of Restoration 234

II. Eden Isn't a Distant Future—It's a Present Invitation 235

III. You Are the Proof Eden Still Matters 236

FINAL PRAYER: A BLESSING FOR THE READER **239**

REFERENCES **241**

THE EDEN WAY TOOLBOX **245**

WHOLE FOOD PLANT-BASED DETOX STARTER PLAN **246**

1. PANTRY PURGE CHECKLIST 246

    Ingredient Red Flags: Get Rid of These *246*

2. BUDGET MEAL PREP 246

3. GENTLE HEALING TOOLS 247

4. REBUILD WITH REAL FOOD 247

5. EDUCATE YOURSELF ON WHOLE FOOD PLANT-BASED BASICS 247

6. STOCK A WFPB-FRIENDLY KITCHEN 248

7. KEEP A FOOD + MOOD JOURNAL 248

8. FOCUS ON SIMPLE, REPEATABLE MEALS 248

9. PREPARE FOR SOCIAL AND EMOTIONAL CHALLENGES 249

10. POTS AND PANS DETOX 249

    Better Alternatives *249*

11. UTENSILS DETOX 250

    Better Alternatives *250*

12. STORAGE CONTAINERS DETOX 250

    Better Alternatives *250*

13. CLEANING TOOLS DETOX 250

    Better Alternatives *251*

EDEN HOME DETOX CHECKLIST **252**

BEDROOM – DETOX FOR REST AND RENEWAL 252

LIVING ROOM – DETOX FOR PEACE AND PRESENCE 252

BATHROOM (ATMOSPHERE FOCUS—BEYOND PRODUCTS) 253

LAUNDRY & ENTRYWAY – DETOX FOR FLOW AND FIRST IMPRESSIONS 253

AIR & LIGHT – DETOX THE ATMOSPHERE ITSELF 254

DIGITAL DETOX ZONES 254

SENSORY PEACE RESET 255

SPIRITUAL ATMOSPHERE 255

RHYTHM & RITUAL DETOX 255

WHOLE-HOME EMOTIONAL RESET 256

PERSONAL CARE DETOX CHECKLIST **257**

1. DEODORANTS 257

Better Alternatives *257*

2.   SHAMPOOS & CONDITIONERS 257

Better Alternatives *257*

3.   LOTIONS & BODY CREAMS 258

Better Alternatives *258*

4.   MAKEUP 258

Better Alternatives *258*

5.   PERFUMES & COLOGNES 259

Better Alternatives *259*

6. BODY WASH & SOAPS 259

Better Alternatives *259*

7-DAY SAMPLE DETOX MENU 260

SCRIPTURES SHOWING YESHUA OPPOSED THE SACRIFICIAL SYSTEM 263

PROPHETIC CHALLENGE TO THE TEMPLE SYSTEM 263

PROPHECIES AGAINST SACRIFICE QUOTED OR LIVED BY YESHUA 264

TEMPLE AND SACRIFICE AS OBSOLETE 264

THE PLOT TO KILL HIM WAS RELIGIOUS, NOT JUST POLITICAL 265

SHABBAT READ ALONG 267

"Shabbat Is Here!" *267*

Write Your Own Psalm Below *268*

EDENIC LIVING BUDGETING WORKSHEET 270

HOW TO USE THIS WORKSHEET 270

MONTHLY INCOME 271

MONTHLY EXPENSES 271

SIMPLICITY AND STEWARDSHIP REFLECTION 272

ABOUT THE AUTHOR 273

Introduction

❦ ❦

Why Not You? Why Not Now?

Do you remember the old adage: you are what you eat? That is quite literally true. Every cell in your body, from your skin to your liver to your brain, is built from the raw materials you provide it. The food you eat becomes your body. Your cells regenerate constantly, and the only building blocks your body has to use are the nutrients (or toxins) you've ingested or stored.

We are made of what we eat—and nothing else. The foods we choose either preserve life or usher in disease. But what if even the so-called healthy foods we're eating are fueling illness instead of healing? What if the "normal" dinner plate includes more than just food? What if it also includes residues of weed killer, bug spray, embalming agents, antibiotics, synthetic dyes, and even arsenic? The truth is sobering: our favorite foods—bananas, cereal, milk, toast—are often laced with substances that were never meant for human consumption.

These toxins build up, lodging deep in our fat cells, our joints, our skin. The body wants to cleanse them, but we never give it the chance. Our body never has the chance to remove them, because we're constantly eating the toxins every day: day-in, day-out. The cycle doesn't stop until we do.

My family and I were caught in that cycle. After three years on a strict keto diet, our health was unraveling. The weight we'd lost had returned, plus more, even though we were strictly following the diet and were deep in ketosis every day. My husband's energy had plummeted, and our daughter gained weight despite eating what was promoted as "clean." As for me, I was exhausted. My weight had yo-yoed most of my life, but now I was dealing with nerve pain, excruciating eczema, Type 2 diabetes, high blood pressure, high cholesterol and triglycerides, and depression. Doctors had no answers, nor were any of the specialists I went to interested in finding the root cause of what was causing my body to break down. I only got more and more prescriptions.

Then came the turning point: a 40-day Daniel Fast. We prayed daily, asking YHVH to show us how to eat for healing, not just survival. The answer came, clear and undeniable: **Return to the beginning. Return to Eden.**

What we discovered is that YHVH's original plan of whole, living, plant-based food was not only the blueprint for health, but a spiritual act of obedience. As we embraced Eden's ways, my husband dropped 70 pounds and felt younger than he had in decades. Our daughter shed the excess weight and gained confidence. I found relief from rashes, clarity of mind, and the gradual reversal of the health conditions that had plagued me.

But here's what surprised me the most: it wasn't just the food that brought healing. It was the alignment. Eden was never just about plants—it was a divine rhythm for all of life. It was a lifestyle of **wholeness**—physical, emotional, and spiritual.

Before there was pain, sickness, or striving—there was Eden. YHVH didn't just place humanity in a garden. He placed them in alignment.

They had:

- Food that healed and sustained (Genesis 1:29)
- Work that was purposeful and life-giving (Genesis 2:15)
- Rest woven into the rhythm of time (Genesis 2:2–3)
- Relationships free from distortion or shame (Genesis 2:25)

- Spiritual intimacy with their Creator, unbroken and daily (Genesis 3:8)

Eden wasn't just a location. It was a design. A blueprint. *A way of being* in harmony with heaven and earth.

That's what we lost.
And that's what we're being called back to.

Tov me'od—"very good" in Hebrew—was the original declaration over mankind. Not just good morally, but wholly functional, beautifully aligned, and bursting with purpose. And while we may not return to Eden in its untouched perfection, we *can* return to its rhythm.

This book isn't just about weight loss or food. It's about freedom. It's about healing. And it's about reclaiming the life we were created for.

I've spent years researching, studying under plant-based pioneers, and trialing nearly every lifestyle out there. I've cried in pain, wrestled in prayer, and watched my family suffer. And I've learned that healing isn't always immediate, but it's always possible.

If you've felt betrayed by your body… if doctors have failed to give you answers… if you've cycled through diets, pills, shame, and desperation—this book is for you. If you've ever asked, "What's wrong with me?" or "Why can't I heal?"—this book will help you reframe that question.

It's not what's wrong with you.

It's what's wrong with what you've been told is *normal.*

Healing doesn't come from hacks. It comes from holiness—or rather, **whole-ness**—in mind, body, and spirit.

But as we return to Eden, we must face an uncomfortable truth: we've forgotten how to walk there.

Eden wasn't just a garden. It was a way of being. A life of alignment, innocence, communion, and purpose. But somewhere along the way, we traded the daily walk with our Creator for disconnection, distraction, and self-reliance. We stopped living in the rhythm we were made for.

James 1:23–24 paints a picture of this forgetfulness:

"For if any one is a hearer of the word and not a doer, he is like unto a man beholding his natural face in a mirror: for he beholdeth himself and goeth away, and straightway forgetteth what manner of man he was."

That's what happened when humanity left Eden. We once saw clearly—made in the image of Elohim, walking with Him in peace and purpose. But when we turned away, we didn't just lose paradise. We lost our sense of self.

James wasn't only speaking of moral drift; he was describing identity loss. We look into the mirror of YHVH's Word and see truth: we are beloved, chosen, designed. But unless we *walk* in that truth, we forget. Not just what to do—but *who we are*.

Returning to Eden isn't about rewinding time. It's about remembering. It's about looking again into the mirror of our design and choosing to live in it. To walk in truth. To embody alignment.

Eden is not just a memory—it's a map.
And the mirror is still there.
So is the Garden.
Let's look—and then live.

Eden is not just a place; it's

A way.

A rhythm.

A return.

We were made for Eden.

So, I invite you to come back to the garden.

Because Eden isn't lost. It's waiting.

And the question isn't, "Will it happen someday?"

The question is,

"Why not now?"

1—Back to the beginning: Why Eden still Matters

❧ ❧

I.   The Blueprint of Eden

Before we ever knew sickness, we were designed for wholeness.

Before there was shame, there was joy.

Before there was fear, there was connection.

Before there was medicine, there was food, and it came from trees.

In Genesis chapters 1 and 2, we find something the world has all but forgotten: a divine pattern. *A blueprint.* This pattern is not just for creation, but for how to live. These chapters aren't mythology. They are medicine for the body, mind, and soul. They are not fantasy. They are a functional health map straight from the Creator of our bodies, minds, and spirits.

The Original Health Plan

When YHVH created mankind, He didn't just place them in a garden. He put them in alignment. Adam and Eve were not designed to manage disease. They were designed to thrive in a perfectly balanced system. The garden supplied everything necessary:

- o Food that healed and sustained (Genesis 1:29)
- o Work that was purposeful and life-giving (Genesis 2:15)
- o Rest woven into the fabric of time (Genesis 2:2–3)
- o Relationships free of distortion or shame (Genesis 2:25)
- o Spiritual intimacy with their Creator, unbroken and daily (Genesis 3:8)

This wasn't just a place to live—it was a design for how to live in harmony with heaven and earth.

Whole, Unashamed, Nourished, Connected

Let's break down these cornerstones, because they still speak to us today:

Whole: The Hebrew mindset doesn't divide the body, soul, and spirit the way modern Western thinking does. Wholeness (shalom) is about integration. It's about being complete, without fragmentation. Adam and Eve didn't need therapy or prescriptions. They were fully present in their bodies, clear in their thoughts, and clean in their hearts.

Unashamed: "They were both naked, the man and his wife, and were not ashamed" (Genesis 2:25). This wasn't just physical nudity. It was emotional transparency. Nothing was hidden. No masks, no fear of judgment. That's the emotional safety we were created for.

Nourished: Genesis 1:29 wasn't a trendy vegan pitch. It was divine provision. Plant-based food was the first prescription, directly from the Creator to His image-bearers. It wasn't just about avoiding meat—it was about consuming life, untouched by death.

Connected: Genesis 3:8 says YHVH walked in the garden with them "in the cool of the day." This wasn't a metaphor. This was intimacy. The presence of YHVH wasn't scheduled or religious—it was relational. They knew Him, and He delighted to be with them.

What Does "Very Good" Actually Mean?

Genesis 1 repeats a rhythm: "And God [Elohim] saw that it was good" (emphasis added). But when mankind is created, the rhythm breaks open into something more profound:

"And God [Elohim] saw everything he had made, and behold, it was **very good**" (Genesis 1:31, emphasis added).

In Hebrew, the phrase is טוֹב מְאֹד (tov me'od). It doesn't just mean "very good." It means exceedingly good, altogether good, intensely and entirely functional, beautiful, and whole.

Tov implies usefulness, benefit, purpose, and harmony.

Me'od amplifies it. It's like turning up the volume to maximum intensity.

YHVH looked at His creation—including mankind—and declared it not just morally good, but completely aligned. Nothing missing. Nothing distorted. Nothing that needed improvement.

The human body was operating in its ideal state. The emotional life was uncluttered. The spiritual connection was direct and unbroken. And every part of creation sang in tune with the Creator's voice.

That's what we lost.

And that's what we're being called back to.

This is why Eden still matters.

Because tov me'od is still possible, not in its original perfection, but in restored alignment, through lifestyle, through obedience, through renewal—we don't have to settle for managing brokenness.

We can pursue wholeness.

And it starts by going back to the beginning.

II.   Four Cornerstones of Edenic Health

~Plant-Based Nourishment

~Purposeful Movement and Stewardship

~ Emotional Integrity

~Spiritual Intimacy

YHVH's design wasn't a list of rules. It was a rhythm.

In Eden, everything worked together. Food wasn't just fuel. Work wasn't just labor. Emotions weren't dangerous. And the spiritual life wasn't a Sunday event. It was a daily walk with the Creator. These four areas formed a complete foundation for whole-being health.

We call them the Four Cornerstones of Edenic Health:

1.   Plant-Based Nourishment

"And God said, Behold, I have given you every herb yielding seed, which is upon the face of all the earth, and every tree, in which is the fruit of a tree yielding seed; to you it shall be for food" Genesis 1:29.

This was the first divine prescription.

Before there were supplements or symptom charts, YHVH gave food directly from the soil. It was unprocessed, alive, and designed for healing.

In the garden, there was no killing. No inflammation. No food allergies. There was just a natural provision that supported the body's design.

Plant-based eating wasn't a fad or a restriction. It was alignment.

9

Every leaf, seed, and fruit were filled with life-giving nutrients, enzymes, fiber, and water. Food didn't just satisfy hunger—it connected Adam and Eve to the land and to their life-giver.

Even today, science is confirming what Genesis made clear:

Plants reduce inflammation. They heal the gut. They feed the brain. They prevent disease. When we eat what we were created for, we don't just feel better—we realign with Eden.

2. Purposeful Movement and Stewardship

"And YHVH God [Elohim] took the man, and put him into the garden of Eden to dress it and to keep it" Genesis 2:15.

The first "job" wasn't about survival. It was about stewardship.

Adam wasn't cursed with work—he was gifted with purpose. He moved his body to cultivate beauty, harvest abundance, and walk in dominion. He wasn't chasing money, burning out, or clocking in. His labor was sacred.

Movement in Eden wasn't punishment. It was part of the joy of being human.

Today, many of us are sedentary, overstressed, and disconnected from our physical purpose. Exercise becomes a chore. Movement becomes shame-based. But in Eden, movement was integrated with meaning.

When we walk, garden, clean, stretch, or move intentionally, we re-enter a divine rhythm. We return to stewardship instead of strain.

3. Emotional Integrity (No Shame, Fear, or Blame)

"And they were both naked, the man and his wife, and were not ashamed" (Genesis 2:25).

This is more than a physical observation. It's an emotional diagnosis.

Before sin, Adam and Eve experienced perfect emotional health. No hiding. No performance. No anxiety. They were fully seen and entirely safe.

But the moment sin entered, so did shame:

- o They covered themselves (Genesis 3:7).
- o They hid from YHVH (v. 8).
- o They blamed each other (v. 12–13).

Emotional fragmentation was one of the first signs of the Fall. And we still carry its scars as defensiveness, insecurity, emotional dysregulation, codependency, and fear of rejection.

In Eden, emotional integrity meant being whole and honest in your soul—no masks, no manipulation, and no fear of being known. That's what we long for. That's what YHVH is restoring.

4. Spiritual Intimacy (Daily Communion with YHVH)

"And they heard the voice of YHVH God walking in the garden in the cool of the day…" (Genesis 3:8).

Before there were temples, Torah scrolls, or priests, there was presence.

YHVH walked with them. Not in fire or thunder, but in the cool of the day.

This was the heart of Eden: unbroken communion with the Creator.

He wasn't far away. He wasn't limited to rituals or buildings. His voice was familiar. His nearness was natural.

Spiritual intimacy wasn't a religious obligation—it was a lifeline.

And though the Fall disrupted that walk, Yeshua the Messiah came to restore it. Through Him, we're invited again into the rhythm of Eden, where YHVH's voice nourishes our spirit, and our days are shaped not by chaos, but by communion.

Eden Was Never Just a Place

It was a pattern.

It held a blueprint for living that nourishes every part of us. And though cherubim and flaming swords guard the garden, the way back is open. It is open through truth, surrender, and the daily choices that realign us with what was…with what *still is* "very good."

These four cornerstones are still available. And they're not optional—they're foundational.

To heal, we don't need to reinvent the wheel.

We need to return to the rhythm.

III.   Why We Long for Eden

There's a quiet ache in the soul of every human being.

It rises not only in our most broken moments, but even in the quiet, ordinary ones:

-when we bite into an apple and somehow still feel empty

-when we cry for no apparent reason

-when we scroll past curated smiles and wonder why joy feels so elusive.

Something in us is always reaching for more. That ache isn't weakness. It's memory. A sacred longing that is encoded for what we were created to experience. We long for Eden because we were designed for Eden. And no amount of modern comfort can erase that truth.

The Ache of Disconnection

Disconnection is the root of almost every symptom we experience in body, mind, and spirit.

We're disconnected from our bodies: treating them like enemies, blaming them for weight gain or fatigue instead of listening to what they're trying to say.

We're disconnected from our emotions: numbing them, resenting them, or letting them rule us without understanding their origin.

We're disconnected from each other: lonely in crowds, guarded in our marriages, and burned out by performance based relationships.

Worst of all, we're disconnected from our Creator: filling our schedules and stomachs but starving our spirits.

This disconnection began in Genesis 3, but it's still alive and well in the 21st century.

We feel it in our inflammation, our anxiety, our depression, our fatigue.

We feel it when we wake up already feeling overwhelmed.

We feel it when we lose our tempers over small things or stay up too late trying to escape reality.

And deep down, we know… this isn't how it's supposed to be.

Eternity Set in Our Hearts

"He hath made everything beautiful in its time: also he hath set eternity in their heart…" Ecclesiastes 3:11.

The Hebrew phrase for "eternity" (ha'olam) implies something both infinite and deeply rooted in the past. It's the sense that we were meant for more. It's the sense that we were meant for timeless connection, enduring peace, and unshakable love. In other words, we were designed with a memory of Eden etched into our very being.

We may not consciously remember walking with YHVH in the cool of the day…

But our souls remember what it felt like to be whole.

And every time we experience pain, loss, or fear, that buried longing whispers:

"Come back."

It's the longing behind our need to belong.

The restlessness behind our constant striving.

The quiet cry behind our health journeys, our therapy sessions, and our prayerful tears.

We don't just want to feel better. We want to go home.

Modern Symptoms of Eden Lost

We don't live in a garden anymore. We live in a whirlwind of blue light, fast food, false identities, and relentless noise. And it's costing us more than we realize.

Here's what Eden *lost* looks like today:

o Processed food that sickens instead of nourishes
o Chronic illness rooted in inflammation, stress, and toxicity
o Mental health crises masked by entertainment and pharmaceuticals
o Spiritual confusion, religious burnout, and counterfeit peace
o Social disconnection, isolation, and distrust
o Perpetual fatigue, decision overwhelm, and identity crisis

We were never meant to live this way. And yet, we normalize dysfunction because it's all we've known.

But inside you—beneath the habits, the trauma, the cravings—there's a spark.

A knowing.

A remembering.

That you were made for more. Not just for heaven one day, but for alignment right here, right now.

IV.   The Good News: Eden Isn't Gone… It's Calling

The gates of the garden were closed after the Fall, but the pattern was never revoked.

Yeshua and the Tree of Life: A Living Teaching

Yeshua revealed the meaning of the Tree of Life not through abstract theology, but by the way He lived, spoke, and invited others into a restored relationship with the Creator. The Tree of Life, first seen in the Garden of Eden, symbolizes divine wisdom, spiritual nourishment, eternal connection, and alignment with YHVH's design. Yeshua embodied these principles in every aspect of His life.

1. He Walked in Perfect Alignment with Torah (Instruction)

Proverbs 3:18 says, "She [wisdom] is a Tree of Life to them that lay hold upon her: And happy is every one that retaineth her" (emphasis added). Yeshua consistently taught and lived out the wisdom of Torah, often quoting directly from it and clarifying its deeper intent. He didn't merely obey YHVH's commandments; he illuminated their meaning at the heart level, encouraging others to go beyond ritual and into relationship. In doing so, He showed that wisdom, rightly applied, leads us back to the Tree of Life.

2. He Offered Living Water and the Bread of Life

In John 4 and 6, Yeshua speaks of living water and bread from heaven, echoing the imagery of Eden where the Tree of Life stood beside the river that nourished the garden. He invited people not just to hear his words, but to internalize them, saying, "…the words that I have spoken unto you are spirit, and are life" (John 6:63). Just as the Tree of Life offered sustaining fruit, Yeshua offered teachings that nourished the soul and brought people back to a place of spiritual vitality.

3. He Modeled the Narrow Path that Leads to Life

In Matthew 7:13–14, Yeshua warned of the broad road that leads to destruction and invited people onto the narrow path that leads to life. This "life" is not just survival or future reward. It is Edenic life:

wholeness, peace (shalom), and intimacy with the Creator. His Sermon on the Mount (Matthew 5–7) is filled with guidance that realigns human behavior, thought, and desire with the Creator's heart.

4. *He Healed and Restored: Physically, Emotionally, Spiritually*

In Eden, the Tree of Life was part of a world without sickness or separation. Yeshua's healing ministry was more than compassion. It was a preview of Eden restored. Every time He healed the sick, forgave sin, or welcomed the outcast, He was revealing what life looks like when it flows from the Tree of Life: wholeness, connection, and freedom.

5. *He Called Us to Abide in Him and Bear Fruit*

In John 15, Yeshua says, "(v.1) I am the true vine, and my Father is the husbandman… (v.5) I am the vine, ye are the branches: he that abideth in me, and I in him, the same beareth much fruit…" This is Eden language. Just as the Tree of Life bore fruit continually, Yeshua invites us to abide in the source of life, to become like fruitful trees ourselves (Psalm 1:3). A life connected to YHVH becomes a life that nourishes others.

Yeshua taught the Tree of Life not as a concept to be worshipped, but as a reality to be lived. Through wisdom, restoration, truth-telling, compassion, and alignment with Torah, He showed us what it means to live a life rooted in the eternal—a life that brings healing to others and leads us back to the Garden.

The ache inside you is not meant to torment you. It's meant to guide you. It's not a signal that you're broken. It's a reminder that you were meant to be whole.

This book is not about returning to an ancient lifestyle out of nostalgia. It's about reclaiming the divine pattern that was written into your design.

You were made for Eden.

And the ache in your soul is your invitation back.

2—The Fall: Root of Disease, Distortion, and Disconnect

☙ ☙

I. What Really Broke in the Garden

To understand healing, we first have to understand the break.

Many of us spend years treating symptoms—eczema, anxiety, inflammation, identity confusion—but never ask the deeper question: Where did this all begin? Why are our bodies turning on themselves? Why do we sabotage what we say we want? Why does peace feel so hard to hold?

The answer isn't modern. It's ancient.

It started not in a hospital... but in a garden.

Not with a diagnosis... but with a decision.

The Turning Point: "Did Elohim Really Say...?"

The serpent's strategy wasn't brute force. It was distortion.

"Now the serpent was more subtle than any beast of the field which JEHOVAH God had made. And he said unto the woman, Yea, hath God said, Ye shall not eat of any tree of the garden," (Genesis 3:1)?

The first temptation wasn't about hunger. It was about trust.

With one question, the enemy planted doubt—about YHVH's word, YHVH's character, and mankind's identity. And with one bite of forbidden fruit, a fracture tore through creation. It wasn't just a bite of food. It was a rejection of design. It was disobedience dressed up as self-improvement.

What Was Lost in One Moment

Genesis 3 gives us the clearest account of what broke.

1. *Food Became a Weapon*

"And when the woman saw that the tree was good for food, and that it was a delight to the eyes, and that the tree was to be desired to make one wise, she took of the fruit thereof, and did eat; and she gave also unto her husband with her, and he did eat" (Genesis 3:6).

The very thing YHVH had used to nourish and sustain was now used in rebellion. Food, once a tool for life, became a tool of deception.

This was the moment food crossed from physical to spiritual. The enemy used appetite to separate humanity from YHVH. And he still does.

Emotional eating, toxic cravings, addiction, and chronic illness all trace back to this disordered relationship with food. We now eat not just for fuel—but to medicate, to escape, to replace the intimacy we lost.

Imagine for a moment someone told you that you could no longer have your favorite food. Think about cherry cheesecake, a cheeseburger, bacon and eggs, steak and potatoes, pizza, ice cream, chocolate cake, or your favorite candy bars…How would you react? That is the power of how appetite and the desire for foods that look good to the eye separates humanity from YHVH.

2. *Shame Was Born*

"And the eyes of them both were opened, and they knew that they were naked; and they sewed fig-leaves together, and made themselves aprons" (Genesis 3:7).

Before the Fall, Adam and Eve were naked and felt no shame. But suddenly, awareness turned into self-consciousness. Intimacy gave way to hiding. Innocence gave way to fear.

Shame is more than embarrassment—it's the fear of being seen. It distorts our relationships, creates emotional strongholds, and becomes the lens through which we interpret our worth. And it began right there in the garden.

3. *Toil Replaced Joy*

"And unto Adam he said, Because thou hast hearkened unto the voice of thy wife, and hast eaten of the tree, of which I commanded thee, saying, Thou shalt not eat of it: cursed is the ground for thy sake; in toil shalt thou eat of it all the days of thy life;" (Genesis 3:17).

Work in Eden *had* been purposeful and joyful. Now, it became survival.

The ground, once generous, turned resistant. Bodies, once energized, turned weary. Burnout and striving were born. The body began aging. The nervous system no longer rested. Hormones began to misfire. Joyful stewardship became painful performance.

We still carry this curse when we work without rest, hustle without purpose, and ignore the divine rhythm of Sabbath.

4. *Separation Entered the Story*

"And they heard the voice of Jehovah God walking in the garden in the cool of the day: and the man and his wife hid themselves from the presence of Jehovah God amongst the trees of the garden," (Genesis 3:8).

This is the most heartbreaking moment in Scripture.

The God who once walked freely with His creation now finds them hiding. They are not running to Him, but from Him. The closeness has fractured.

And that fracture still defines much of our spiritual experience: distance, silence, guilt, disconnection. We search for intimacy with YHVH, but we feel unworthy. We perform instead of commune. We beg instead of abide.

This was not how it was meant to be.

The High Cost of Disobedience

Disobedience didn't just break a rule. It broke relationship. It disrupted alignment. It polluted the body, confused the mind, destabilized emotions, and severed the spiritual lifeline.

The cost was:

- o Physical suffering
- o Emotional fragmentation
- o Relational conflict
- o Spiritual exile

And we see the effects in every hospital room, every anxious mind, every broken marriage, every confused soul.

But the Story Didn't End There

Even in judgment, YHVH moved with mercy:

> ~He clothed their shame (Genesis 3:21).

> ~`He promised a Deliverer (Genesis 3:15).

He removed them from the garden not to punish—but to prevent eternal separation through the Tree of Life (Genesis 3:22–24).

What broke in the garden—food, trust, identity, intimacy—is exactly what Yeshua messiah came to restore.

But first, we have to understand the fracture…

So, we can follow the Way back to wholeness.

II. The Threefold Death

When YHVH warned Adam, "…for in the day that thou eatest thereof thou shalt surely die" (Genesis 2:17), it's easy to assume death meant only the end of physical life. But Adam didn't fall over dead the moment he bit into the fruit.

Something more complex and far-reaching happened.

Death did come—but it came in three layers, each one fracturing a different part of humanity's design.

This is the Threefold Death: physical, emotional, and spiritual. And it explains why we feel broken on so many levels—why we can exercise and still feel anxious, why we can go to church and still feel numb, why we can eat healthy and still get sick.

The Fall didn't just wound one part of us—it wounded all three.

1. Physical Death: Disease, Aging, and the Decay of the Body

Before the Fall, the human body was not designed to die. It was designed to live in unbroken rhythm with creation and the Creator. There was no inflammation, no insulin resistance, no arthritis or autoimmune disease. Food was perfect. The environment was clean. The nervous system was calm.

But sin introduced stress, fear, sweat, and struggle. The ground was cursed. The body, once sustained by divine design, began to deteriorate.

"In the sweat of thy face shalt thou eat bread, till thou return unto the ground; for out of it wast thou taken: for dust thou are, and unto dust shalt thou return" (Genesis 3:19).

Every wrinkle, every ache, every chronic condition is evidence of this physical decay. Even the healthiest among us will age. The body now carries the sentence of mortality.

But it's not just death at the end of life—it's the slow death we experience in our cells every day:

Chronic inflammation

Hormonal disruption

Nutritional deficiencies

Gut breakdown

Genetic mutations

Modern disease is a symptom of ancient disobedience.

But through obedience and alignment, we can slow the decay and restore function—even if we can't yet eliminate death itself.

2. Emotional Death: Shame, Fear, and Blame

The moment Adam and Eve sinned, their emotional landscape shifted.

"And the eyes of them both were opened, and they knew that they were naked; and they sewed fig-leaves together, and made themselves aprons" (Genesis 3:7).

"And he [Adam] said, I heard thy voice in the garden, and I was afraid, because I was naked; and I hid myself" (Genesis 3:10, emphasis added).

Before the Fall, there was emotional wholeness—no self-consciousness, no insecurity, no relational tension. But now:

Innocence was replaced with shame.

Confidence was replaced by fear.

Responsibility was replaced by blame.

These emotional responses weren't just behavioral—they were neurological and spiritual breakdowns. The nervous system that once operated in peace now lived in fight-or-flight mode.

We still carry these patterns today:

People-pleasing and perfectionism (shame)

Social anxiety and panic (fear)

Defensiveness and bitterness (blame)

These emotional reflexes are inherited defaults—strongholds we must intentionally dismantle. Because until we deal with emotional death, we will keep sabotaging physical and spiritual healing.

3. Spiritual Death: Disconnection from YHVH

The most devastating consequence of the Fall wasn't sickness or shame. It was separation.

"Therefore, Jehovah God sent him [Adam] forth from the garden of Eden, to till the ground from whence he was taken," (Genesis 3:23, emphasis added).

Before the Fall, Adam and Eve had face-to-face communion with their Creator. Afterward, that connection was severed. The Tree of Life was no longer accessible. The presence of YHVH became something feared instead of cherished.

Spiritual death is the root of every other form of death.

Because without the Source, there can be no sustained healing.

We were created to walk with YHVH, not just obey Him. To hear His voice, not just follow His rules. To rest in His love, not perform for acceptance. But sin drove a wedge between us and the One who sustains our very breath.

This spiritual disconnection still plays out today:

> We perform instead of abide.

> We fear punishment instead of trust His heart.

> We seek meaning everywhere except in Him.

The ultimate consequence of the Fall is this:

We lost access to the only One who can restore us.

Why the Threefold Death Matters

If we try to fix physical symptoms without addressing spiritual disconnection, healing will be shallow.

If we treat emotional triggers without changing the lies we believe, the patterns will return.

If we seek spiritual growth without nourishing the body or renewing the mind, we'll burn out.

The Threefold Death requires a threefold restoration.

That's what this book is about.

We must:

1. Restore the body through obedience to the Creator's design.

2. Heal the mind and emotions through truth, repentance, and identity realignment.

3. Reconnect with YHVH through intimacy, rest, and daily communion

Only then can we experience the kind of shalom that Eden once held.

III. Generational Patterns and Modern Manifestations

The effects of the Fall didn't end with Adam and Eve.

Their choices set into motion a ripple of consequences that would affect every human being after them: emotionally, physically, and spiritually. These weren't isolated consequences. They became patterns.

They became wounds passed down from generation to generation.

We carry them in our bodies.

We echo them in our thoughts.

We repeat them in our families and communities.

And until we name them for what they are, we'll keep living under their weight without even realizing why.

The Torah Shows the Pattern of Inheritance

Throughout the Scriptures, we see a clear theme: the actions of one generation affect the next.

Adam and Eve's disobedience opened the door to death and toil—not just for themselves, but for their children.

Cain inherited the struggle and became the first murderer.

Generational consequences show up repeatedly, such as in Exodus 20:5, where YHVH warns that iniquity can affect children "to the third and fourth generation."

This isn't about punishment—it's about pattern. When sin, trauma, or disconnection isn't healed, it gets passed down.

Today, we experience that inheritance in our genetics, our nervous systems, *and* our belief systems. Ancient disobedience has become modern dysfunction.

1 Inherited Trauma: The Emotional Echo of Eden's Loss

You don't have to live through a war or a tragedy to carry trauma.

Sometimes, it lives in the family atmosphere you grew up in. Sometimes, it's passed down in silence, fear, or control.

When Adam and Eve hid from YHVH in shame, they taught us that hiding is safer than healing.

When blame entered the relationship between Adam and Eve, it modeled distrust and defensiveness.

When Cain reacted in anger and isolation, he showed what happens when wounds go unprocessed.

This emotional inheritance still shows up today in:

> Fear of intimacy,

> Control and perfectionism,

> Emotional shutdown or explosive reactions,

> Cycles of mistrust, bitterness, and unworthiness.

These aren't just personality quirks—they're echoes of Eden lost.

2 Chronic Inflammation: The Physical Manifestation of Disconnection

From the moment the ground was cursed and labor became toil, the human body began to suffer under strain.

We now live with physical symptoms that are rooted not just in diet, but in disorder—disorder in our rhythms, disorder in our beliefs, disorder in our environment.

Inflammation is a key manifestation of this disorder. It fuels:

> Autoimmune disease

Heart conditions

Gut dysfunction

Mood imbalances

Hormonal chaos

Stress and disconnection pour fuel on the fire. When we live in a state of constant alert—emotionally or spiritually—our bodies follow suit.

YHVH's design was for rest, peace, nourishment, and trust. When we operate outside of that design, our bodies bear the burden.

3 Identity Confusion: The Mental Fog of a Fractured Design

One of the first signs of the Fall was identity distortion. Adam and Eve went from walking confidently with YHVH to hiding from Him. They began covering themselves and distancing from one another. That distortion has grown over time.

In our generation, identity confusion is rampant:

People define themselves by their trauma instead of their Creator.

Value is tied to performance, appearance, or comparison.

Gender, purpose, and belonging are questioned at foundational levels.

When we don't know who we are, we will look everywhere—culture, emotion, even pain—for answers. But we were never meant to self-define. We were meant to reflect the image of the One who made us.

The further we drift from Eden, the harder it is to remember who we really are.

Breaking the Pattern

The good news is: what has been inherited can be interrupted.

YHVH never leaves His people without hope. Over and over again, He calls us to return, to remember, to realign. He offers blessings for obedience and healing for those who walk in His ways.

"See, I have set before thee this day life and good, and death and evil; [19]I call heaven and earth to witness against you this day, that I have set before thee life and death, the blessing and the curse: therefore, choose life, that thou mayest life, thou and they seed;" (Deuteronomy 30:15,19).

You are not bound to repeat what you were born into.

You are not doomed to carry the same inflammation, the same emotional wounds, or the same spiritual confusion as your ancestors.

Through repentance, restoration, and realignment with the Creator's design, you can reset the pattern.

You can restore what was broken.

You can be the generation that turns the story around.

IV. Hope Foreshadowed

Even in the moment of exile, YHVH moved with compassion.

The Fall brought disobedience, death, shame, and separation—but the story didn't end with a curse. From the very beginning, YHVH wove hope into the aftermath. And through subtle, powerful signs in Genesis 3, He pointed to something greater: restoration.

Garments of Grace

"And Jehovah God made for Adam and his wife coats of skins, and clothed them" (Genesis 3:21).

In a moment dripping with mercy, YHVH provided covering.

Adam and Eve had tried to cover themselves with fig leaves—hastily stitched, fragile attempts to hide their shame. But it wasn't enough. They needed something more durable, something that came from YHVH's own hands.

These garments of skin were not a punishment—they were an act of grace. The Hebrew word for "skin," ʿôr, (עוֹר) can also carry connotations of protection, boundary, and new identity. It symbolized YHVH's ongoing care, even after discipline.

This was not the beginning of religious ritual. This was the Creator saying: You may be leaving the garden, but you are not leaving My care.

Today, we still try to cover ourselves with performance, perfectionism, and self-made solutions. But healing never comes from fig leaves. It comes from truth, surrender, and the divine covering of grace.

The Promise of Restoration

"And I will put enmity between thee and the woman, and between thy seed and her seed: he shall bruise thy head, and thou shalt bruise his heel," (Genesis 3:15).

This verse, spoken directly to the serpent, holds the first prophetic hint of restoration.

The "seed of the woman" would rise up—not as a violent conqueror, but as an humble, powerful, Spirit-filled man who would crush the head of the deceiver and expose the lies that fractured creation. His heel would be bruised— yes, but the serpent's dominion would be undone.

This wasn't a promise of blood payment.

It was a promise of reversal.

Of return.

Of renewal.

Messiah: The One Who Laid Down His Life to End Death's Reign

Yeshua didn't come to uphold the system of sacrifice. He came to confront it.

He walked into a world where animals were still being slaughtered in the name of atonement—a system that YHVH never even wanted (Psalm 40:6-8, 51:16-17, Hosea 6:6, Matthew 9:13, Isaiah 1:11-17). Yeshua's mission was not to become a substitute for sin, but to end the cycle of death, violence, and distorted worship.

He was murdered—not as a cosmic transaction—but because He challenged the power structures that upheld spiritual blindness and religious corruption. And He chose that path, willingly laying down His life.

"No one taketh it away from me, but I lay it down of myself…" (John 10:18).

He stood in the place where innocent animals had long been placed, not to legitimize the system, but to dismantle it with love, truth, and obedience to YHVH.

Through His death, the veil was torn. Not because He was a required sacrifice, but because He revealed the heart of the Father—a heart that has always longed for mercy, not sacrifice, (Hosea 6:6).

*For more details: The Eden Way Toolkit: Scriptures Showing Yeshua Opposed the Sacrificial System.

The Garden Was Closed—But the Way Was Not Lost

Even as Adam and Eve stepped outside Eden, the promise of return was already stirring.

Through garments of grace, YHVH showed compassion.

Through prophecy, He pointed to a liberator.

Through the life and death of Yeshua, that promise came into focus— not as a legal transaction, but as an invitation to realign with the Creator's original design.

Hope was never about escaping to heaven. It was about the restoration of what was lost:

Peace. Wholeness. Intimacy. Eden.

3—The Garden Diet: Why Food is Spiritual

I. Food as Divine Assignment

Before there were cravings, diets, or debates about macros and calories, there was a garden. And in that garden, food wasn't a problem to solve—it was a gift to receive.

"Then Elohim said, 'Behold, I have given you every seed-bearing plant on the face of the whole earth and every tree that has fruit with seed in it. They will be yours for food'," (Genesis 1:29).

This verse isn't just about nutrition. It is a divine assignment—the very first instruction YHVH gave humanity regarding their relationship with the earth, their bodies, and their Creator. And it was centered around plants.

The Edenic diet wasn't random. It was sacred.

It was not merely permission—it was direction.

Food as a Sacred Starting Point

YHVH could have begun His relationship with mankind in a thousand ways. He could have started with a list of moral laws, a system of worship, or a blueprint for civilization.

But He began with food.

Why? Because food is fundamental. It shapes our biology, our behavior, our rhythms, and our relationships. What we eat determines how we feel, think, act, and connect—not just with others, but with YHVH Himself.

In Eden, food was not just for survival. It was a daily communion with the land and the One who made it. To eat from the trees was to participate in the ongoing provision and beauty of the Creator. To nourish the body was to honor the design.

The Edenic Diet: Plant-Based and Blood-Free

Genesis 1:29 makes it clear: the original diet was entirely plant-based. Seed-bearing plants and fruit-bearing trees were humanity's intended nourishment. There was no animal flesh. No slaughter. No death was required to sustain life.

This was no accident. It reflected the values of YHVH and of Eden itself:

Life over death

Harmony over violence

Sufficiency without exploitation

Food was to come from what could be freely gathered, not what had to be hunted or killed. In Eden, eating was not a participation in bloodshed—it was an act of gratitude and obedience.

It wasn't until after the Fall—and then again after the flood—that meat entered the human diet. But in the beginning, in the garden, the Creator gave food that brought life without taking it.

Eating as Worship and Obedience

Every bite in Eden was worship.

Not because it was ritualized, but because it was aligned.

To receive what YHVH had provided in the way He provided it was an act of trust. Adam and Eve didn't need to question food labels, count nutrients, or avoid toxins. What they ate reflected their relationship with YHVH—simple, pure, and obedient.

Contrast that with what caused their fall: eating something YHVH told them not to eat.

The first sin wasn't stealing or violence. It was a dietary rebellion—a bite rooted in deception and desire.

That alone tells us how deeply spiritual food truly is.

When we eat in alignment with YHVH's instruction, we reflect trust and stewardship.

When we eat in rebellion or indulgence, we mimic the pattern that broke the world.

This doesn't mean food must be feared—it means it must be respected.

The Daily Choice to Align or Depart

Even now, every meal is a moment of decision.

We can eat in agreement with life, or in accord with the culture of death.

We can choose food that heals or food that harms.

We can draw close to YHVH by honoring His design—or drift away by ignoring it.

Food is not neutral. It never was.

In Eden, it was a tool for connection.

After the Fall, it became a battleground.

Now, it is an invitation—back to the garden rhythm.

II. The Spiritual Weight of Eating

We often separate the physical from the spiritual, as if eating is a purely bodily function and holiness is reserved for prayer. But in Scripture, there's no such divide. Food is spiritual. What we consume is not just about health—it's about alignment.

From Eden to Sinai, from the prophets to the early assemblies, eating has always carried weight, not just in our bodies, but in our relationship with YHVH.

Leviticus Food Laws: Discernment, Holiness, and Vitality

In Leviticus 11 and Deuteronomy 14, YHVH gives detailed instructions on what animals are clean and unclean for consumption. At first glance, these may seem arbitrary or ceremonial. However, a deeper look reveals something sacred: discernment, separation, and protection of life.

"For I am Jehovah your God: sanctify yourselves therefore, and be ye holy; for I am holy: neither shall ye defile yourselves with any manner of creeping thing that moveth upon the earth," (Leviticus 11:44).

Why did YHVH care about food? He cared, because He was teaching

His people to distinguish between what brings life and what leads to corruption.

These dietary instructions were not about rigid religion. They were a form of daily spiritual training—learning to pause, to ask, to obey. Eating became a moment to choose obedience over appetite, wisdom over impulse, trust over convenience.

Even biologically, these laws promoted vitality:

> Clean animals were less likely to carry parasites or toxins.

> Forbidden creatures like pigs and shellfish are nature's filters—designed to clean, not be consumed.

> Obedience protected not just the soul, but the body.

The message was clear: what you eat either honors life or invites decay.

Acts 15: Food and the Gentile Believers

When non-Jewish followers of the Messiah began entering the faith in the first century, the early apostles faced a decision: What parts of the Torah were essential for them to walk in truth and fellowship?

In Acts 15, we see the apostles agree on a foundational starting point:

"... that ye abstain from things sacrificed to idols, and from blood, and from things strangled, and from fornication; from which if ye keep yourselves, it shall be well with you. Fare ye well," (Acts 15:29).

This was not the abolishment of Torah—it was the entry point for Gentiles learning to walk in holiness.

Notice what's included:

> No idolatry,

No blood consumption,

No eating animals that weren't properly drained of blood (strangled).

These were basic food instructions rooted in Leviticus. They weren't about tradition. They were about respecting life, honoring boundaries, and walking in agreement with YHVH's values.

Food mattered then. And it still does now.

Why YHVH Cares What We Eat

YHVH doesn't give instructions because He's controlling. He gives them because He's a Designer, and He knows what our bodies—and spirits—need to thrive.

He made us.

He knows what fuels healing and what fosters harm.

He knows how trauma lives in our gut, how inflammation affects our mind, how blood carries life.

To the Creator, food is not just fuel. It's a touchpoint for:

Obedience — Will we eat what He has provided or what the world markets?

Holiness — Will we be set apart in our kitchens and choices?

Trust — Will we believe He knows better than our cravings?

We live in a culture where food is entertainment, addiction, distraction, and rebellion. But in YHVH's economy, food is sacred. Every meal is an opportunity to align with life—or to drift toward death.

Eating as a Form of Worship

Worship is not just singing songs—it's the daily act of aligning our lives with YHVH's ways. When we choose food that gives life, honors the body, and reflects the values of Eden, we worship.

Choosing whole, plant-based nourishment is a return to Eden.

Avoiding blood, unclean meats, and processed toxins is a return to holiness.

Blessing our food, preparing it with intention, and sharing it in peace is a return to covenant.

Food is not just a private choice. It's a visible expression of what we believe about the Creator—and about ourselves.

III. Blood, Life, and the Heart of the Father

From the beginning, Scripture teaches us that blood is sacred. It is not a flavor enhancer. It is not a culinary tradition. It is life itself.

"For the life of the flesh is in the blood…" (Leviticus 17:11).

Blood belongs to YHVH. And throughout the Torah, we are repeatedly instructed not to consume it. Why? Because it represents life, something only the Creator can give and take. It is not meant for human consumption. And though some have tried to follow the law by "draining" blood from meat, science and common sense both confirm what Scripture already implies:

You cannot remove all the blood from the flesh of an animal.

41

The Body Is Bathed in Blood—Every Cell, Every Fiber

From the moment a heart begins to beat, blood flows through every vessel, carrying oxygen, nutrients, hormones, and life-sustaining messages to the entire body. It does not simply flow through large veins; it moves into the tiniest capillaries, bathing every organ, every muscle, every fiber, and every cell.

Blood travels to microscopic vessels so small they can only carry red blood cells in single file.

It nourishes bones, joints, intestines, skin, and even fat.

It is not stored in one part of the body—it is the circulatory life force *of* the body.

Even when an animal is "bled out," large pools of blood may be removed, but what remains is soaked deep into tissues and cells, impossible to extract.

To consume the flesh is, unavoidably, to consume the blood. And to consume the blood is, according to Scripture, to consume life that does not belong to us.

The Prohibition of Blood Consumption

YHVH's command to abstain from blood is one of the clearest dietary instructions in all of Scripture:

"But flesh with the life thereof, *which is* the blood thereof, shall ye not eat," (Genesis 9:4).

"For as to the life of all flesh, the blood thereof is *all one* with the life thereof: therefore, I said unto the children of Israel, Ye shall eat the blood of no manner of flesh; for the life of all flesh is the blood thereof: whosoever eateth it shall be cut off," (Leviticus 17:14).

"Only be sure that thou eat not the blood: for the blood is the life; and thou shalt not eat the life with the flesh," (Deuteronomy 12:23).

This command was not cultural. It was moral and spiritual.

Blood was never meant to be ingested—it was to be honored. To consume it, even unintentionally, is to cross a sacred line. It symbolically—and biologically—unites us with death.

Animal Death Post-Fall: A Mercy and a Consequence

In Eden, there was no death. The human diet was plant-based. The environment was one of peace. But after sin entered, death followed— and not just for humans.

When Adam and Eve tried to cover their shame with fig leaves, YHVH did something profound:

"And Jehovah God made for Adam and for his wife coats of skins, and clothed them," (Genesis 3:21).

This was the first recorded death of an animal in Scripture. It was an act of mercy—covering their vulnerability. But it was also a consequence of disobedience.

Animal death became a temporary allowance in a world no longer aligned with Eden. It was never the ideal. And while sacrifices would become part of religious life, YHVH never wanted them.

The prophets cried out:

"For I desire goodness, and not sacrifice; and the knowledge of God more than burnt-offerings," (Hosea 6:6).

Yeshua's Teachings on the Restoration of Life

Yeshua, like the prophet Jeremiah before him, did not come to uphold or glorify the temple's system of slaughter. He came to expose the distortion it had become—and to point people back to the Father's original heart: life, not death; obedience, not ritual; restoration, not repetition. (For more details: The Eden Way Toolkit: Scriptures Showing Yeshua Opposed the Sacrificial System)

He taught that true life comes through:

> Trust in the Father,

> Loving one another,

> Returning to righteousness,

> Walking in the light,

> Feeding the hungry, healing the broken, and setting captives free.

"I came that they may have life, and may have *it* abundantly," (John 10:10).

Yeshua willingly laid down His life, not as a sacrificial payment to appease wrath, but as an act of protest against violence, hypocrisy, and corrupted religion. His teachings exposed the false peace of the temple system and invited us back into the shalom of Eden.

Human hands shed his blood—but His message was one of healing, not appeasement. His life revealed that restoration doesn't come through more death—it comes through alignment with truth.

The Heart of the Father Has Always Been Life

YHVH's instructions around blood were not about control—they were about connection. He was teaching His people that life is sacred, and that they were created to honor, not consume, that life.

When we abstain from blood, we declare that life is not ours to take lightly.

When we reject violence and choose peace in our diet, we return to Edenic values.

When we embrace Yeshua's teachings, we reclaim the path to wholeness—not through death, but through obedient living.

You were not designed for a death culture.

You were created for life—pure, sacred, whole.

And every meal is a chance to agree with the heart of the Father.

IV. Eating as Alignment

Food is never just about food.

Every bite is a statement. Every meal is a choice—either toward life or toward disease, toward alignment or toward disconnection. And Scripture makes this clear:

"I call heaven and earth to witness against you this day, that I have set before thee life and death, the blessing and the curse: therefore, choose life, that thou mayest live, thou and thy seed;" (Deuteronomy 30:19).

Choosing life is not only a moral or spiritual decision. It's a physical one.

What we put on our plates is either a vote for the Creator's design or a submission to the world's distortions.

Eating in alignment with Eden is a form of repentance—a return, a turning away from manmade convenience and back toward divine wisdom.

Eating as a Spiritual Act of Alignment

In the modern world, food has been reduced to numbers—calories, macros, points. But in Scripture, food is sacred. It's tied to obedience, covenant, community, and worship.

In Eden, food was the first assignment.

After the Fall, it became the first act of rebellion.

Now, it remains a daily opportunity to recalibrate our alignment with YHVH.

> When we choose foods that:
>
> Grow from the ground,
>
> Come without blood,
>
> Are consumed with gratitude and mindfulness, we're not just nourishing our bodies—we're returning to our design.

Obedience doesn't have to be loud. Sometimes, it looks like a bowl of lentils, a cup of herbal tea, or a clean plate prepared with peace and purpose.

Healing the Gut—and the Soul—With Edenic Food

Modern science is confirming what Torah wisdom has modeled for millennia: the gut is central to human health. Roughly 70% of the immune system resides in the gut (Belkaid, 2017). The gut and brain communicate through the vagus nerve, forming the gut-brain axis, which impacts not only digestion but also mental and emotional health (Mayer, 2015). Additionally, gut microbes influence the production of neurotransmitters, hormones, and inflammatory responses (Cryan, 2019).

But processed food, inflammatory oils, and animal-based diets often disrupt gut health, leading to dysbiosis, leaky gut, and chronic inflammation (Tilg, 2020).

Edenic food, by contrast, is restorative:

> Fiber-rich plants promote microbial diversity and feed beneficial bacteria.

> Fruits and vegetables soothe inflammation and support detoxification.

> Whole grains and legumes provide prebiotics and support metabolic balance.

And healing extends beyond the gut. When we eat in peace—foods designed by YHVH, prepared without violence, and consumed in gratitude—we restore more than the digestive tract. We restore shalom—the wholeness of body, mind, and spirit.

The Daily Return

Every day you eat is a day you get to return.

Return, not just to health, but to harmony between body, soul, and Spirit.

Between you and creation.

Between you and your Creator.

You're not just feeding hunger. You're feeding identity, purpose, and connection.

You don't need a perfect diet.

You need alignment.

And that begins with honoring the wisdom YHVH embedded in the earth and in your own body.

You were made for Eden. And Eden is not just a memory—it's a model.

4—The Silent Saboteurs: Hidden Poisons in Modern Food

❧❧

I. The Chemistry of Compromise

Edenic food was clean, nourishing, and free from human tampering. Today, the grocery store is a minefield of compromise. Common additives like monosodium glutamate (MSG), artificial dyes (such as Red 40), preservatives (like BHA and BHT), and emulsifiers (like polysorbates) disrupt cellular function and inflame the body. High-fructose corn syrup and ultra-processed seed oils (e.g., soybean and canola) have been linked to obesity, insulin resistance, and fatty liver disease. Even "natural flavors"—a deceptive label—can include hidden allergens or excitotoxins.

Scientific studies confirm the damage: these ingredients contribute to chronic inflammation, gut dysbiosis, hormonal imbalance, and mood disorders.

II. Spiritual Consequences of Eating What Was Never Food

Food is meant to nourish both body and soul—it is a form of covenant with the Creator. When we consume chemically engineered substances that hijack our taste buds and damage our bodies, we violate the sacred act of nourishment. Many of these substances are addictive, acting like pharmakeia—substances that dull our senses, cloud discernment, and enslave us.

Choosing to detox from these foods is more than a health decision. It is an act of spiritual repentance and a declaration of war against the systems of Babylon. By refusing these silent saboteurs, we honor YHVH with our bodies.

III. From Slavery to Stewardship

Modern food corporations have engineered products for addiction—combining sugar, salt, and fat in ratios that trigger dopamine release and override natural fullness signals. Like Egypt enslaved the Israelites with brick quotas and harsh labor, processed food enslaves modern minds with craving cycles and chronic illness.

Freedom begins with discernment. Learning to read labels, choosing whole-food alternatives, and praying over what we consume allows us to reclaim our role as stewards, not slaves.

V.   Creating a Detox Plan

Here are four powerful steps to begin your food detox.

Pantry Purge

Remove items with artificial dyes, seed oils, added sugars, MSG, and synthetic preservatives.

Budget Meal Prep

Make large batches of soups, beans, whole grains, and Edenic salads with seasonal produce.

Gentle Healing Tools

Hydration, herbal teas (like dandelion and nettle), and high-fiber foods like chia, flax, and vegetables support elimination.

Rebuild with Real Food

After clearing out and cleansing, nourish your body with vibrant, whole foods. Focus on fresh fruits, raw and steamed vegetables, sprouted legumes, soaked nuts and seeds, and fermented foods like sauerkraut or coconut yogurt. These replenish your gut, rebalance your microbiome, and realign your body with the Creator's design for nourishment.

*See The Eden Way Toolbox at the back of the book for a checklist.

*See the Eden Way Tool Box for a 7-Day Sample Detox Menu.

VI. When the Vessel Poisons the Offering: Toxins in Cookware and Storage

Even when we fill our plates with Edenic foods, the containers we cook and store them in can sabotage their purity. Plastic utensils, food storage bags, and non-stick cookware often leach toxic chemicals, especially when exposed to heat, oil, or acidic foods.

Plastic Storage Containers and Utensils

Plastics marked BPA-free often contain substitute chemicals like BPS and BPF, which research now shows may be just as harmful. These endocrine disruptors mimic hormones, interfere with fertility, disrupt thyroid function, and have been linked to early puberty, metabolic issues, and breast cancer risk. Heating plastic—even in the microwave or dishwasher—accelerates this leaching.

Aluminum Cookware

Though lightweight and affordable, aluminum is a neurotoxin that can leach into food, especially when cooking acidic ingredients like tomatoes or citrus. Studies have connected elevated aluminum exposure with cognitive decline and neurodegenerative disorders such as Alzheimer's disease.

Copper Cookware

Unlined copper pots and pans can leach toxic levels of copper into food during cooking. Excess copper in the diet has been associated with liver damage, gastrointestinal distress, and mineral imbalances.

While some cookware is lined with stainless steel, wear and tear can expose the copper beneath over time.

"Thou shalt not offer the blood of my sacrifice with leavened bread; neither shall the fat of my feast remain all night until the morning" Exodus 23:18.

Even in the details of how offerings were prepared, purity was paramount. Should we offer our meals to YHVH with compromised vessels?

*See The Eden Way Toolbox at the back of the book for a checklist.

Safer Alternatives

Choosing cookware made from glass, cast iron, stainless steel, or ceramic-coated materials ensures that what starts as a nourishing offering remains uncontaminated. Food-grade silicone bags and beeswax wraps can replace plastic for storage, keeping both your body and the environment safe.

The spiritual parallel is clear: even the most righteous food can be tainted by unclean vessels. In the same way, truth can be distorted by the medium that carries it. Returning to the Creator's design means examining every level of what we consume—not just the ingredient list, but the bowl it's served in.

*For a checklist on safe utensils, cookware, and storage containers, see The Eden Way Tool Box at the back of this book.

5—Undoing Babylon: Escaping the Lies of Modern Wellness

I. Recognizing Babylon's Influence

If Eden represents order, peace, and wholeness, Babylon represents the opposite: confusion, exploitation, and falsehood all dressed up in a garment of brilliance. While YHVH designed Eden to bring life, Babylon is the system that distorts that life at every level—physically, emotionally, mentally, and spiritually.

"And I heard another voice from heaven, saying, 'Come forth, my people, out of her, that ye have no fellowship with her sins, and that ye receive not of her plagues:'" (Revelation 18:4).

Babylon is not just a city—it's a spiritual system. A mindset. A way of life that infiltrates our choices, including how we pursue health. And it's become the foundation of much of what we now call "wellness."

Confusion: The Signature of Babylon

The Hebrew word Bavel (בָּבֶל), aka Babylon, comes from the root balal (בָּלַל), which means to mix, to confuse, to mingle what should remain distinct. Babylon thrives where boundaries blur:

> Clean and unclean

> Truth and trend

> Healing and harm.

Modern wellness mirrors this confusion. One moment, fat is evil; the next, it's holy. One decade says "count calories," the next says "ignore them." We are constantly bombarded with mixed messages, health fads, influencer tips, and industry-funded research that leaves us exhausted, overwhelmed, and still sick.

This isn't random. It's the system doing exactly what Babylon does best: creating confusion so that we lose the clarity YHVH intended.

Excess: When "More" Becomes the Disease

In Eden, everything was enough. There was abundance without excess. Simplicity without lack. But Babylon whispers the lie that more is always better—more protein, more supplements, more testing, more restriction, more money spent in the name of "health."

We now live in a culture where:

> Diets sell identity.

> Exercise becomes a punishment.

> Wellness is marketed as a luxury lifestyle.

"Clean" products are mass-produced with hidden toxins.

Body perfection is chased, while peace is sacrificed.

This is not wellness. This is bondage in disguise. Babylon takes the sacred and makes it strife-filled. It turns stewardship into performance and healing into hustle.

Performance: The Disguised Idol of Modern Health

At the heart of Babylon is self-glorification. It builds towers, monuments, and images that say, "Look at me." Modern wellness has absorbed this spirit. Health is no longer about restoration—it's about achievement.

"Fitspiration" replaces joy with judgment.

Clean eating becomes a measure of worthiness.

Social media turns health into a highlight reel.

We are taught to obsess over how we look, rather than how we function. To chase external control while neglecting internal wholeness. We perform for approval from strangers instead of listening to our bodies and honoring our Creator.

This is not Eden. This is Babylon with a green smoothie in hand.

Pharmakeia: The False Priesthood of Healing

"...for with thy sorcery were all the nations deceived," (Revelation 18:23).

The Greek word pharmakeia (φαρμακεία), used here, is translated "sorcery," but it also refers to the mixing of potions, drug-based control, and false healing systems. Babylon's influence is most dangerous when it masquerades as medicine.

This isn't a condemnation of all medical care—many interventions are life-saving. However, much of what we call healthcare today is profit-driven symptom management. ***It is not healing.*** The system thrives on dependency, not restoration.

> Drugs that mask rather than correct.

> Procedures that profit rather than prevent.

> Diagnoses that define rather than free.

> Drugs that cause side effects which are then treated with more drugs to address the side effects.

It's a vicious, insane cycle of decay. Babylon builds temples of white coats and insurance codes. It offers a false sense of peace in the form of a pill or a prescription, often without addressing or even seeking the root cause.

And worse, it conditions people to ignore the body's signals and surrender authority to institutions instead of the Creator.

Counterfeit Healing and False Peace

Babylon doesn't heal—it hides. It distracts. It medicates. It replaces repentance with performance, rest with supplements, and connection with control.

This is the lie we must escape.

True healing doesn't require us to worship our bodies, obsess over metrics, or chase the latest trend. It calls us back to truth, simplicity, obedience, and trust in YHVH's design.

The more we walk in the ways of Babylon, the more disoriented, disconnected, and dependent we become.

But the moment we stop, pause, and ask: Is this Eden or is this empire? We begin the return.

II. Diet Culture vs. Edenic Culture

When you hear the word "diet," what rises up in you? Freedom or fear?

In modern culture, diets are not about nourishment. They are about control. They're driven by image, restriction, marketing, and shame. But the Edenic way is entirely different. It isn't focused on weight loss, punishment, or perfection—it's focused on life.

The Creator never meant for food to torment us. He meant for it to nourish, align, and restore. And when we contrast the world's diet culture with YHVH's Edenic rhythm, the difference couldn't be more evident.

Shame-Based Restrictions vs. Creator-Based Nourishment

Diet culture thrives on shame. It tells you:

> "You are not enough."

> "You must earn your worth."

> "You must shrink yourself to be loved."

It labels food as "good" or "bad," attaches morality to your plate, and makes you fear your appetite. And when you inevitably "fail" the diet, it offers you a new one… with the same bondage, repackaged.

But in Eden, food was not about shame. It was about trust.

"And God said, Behold, I have given you every herb yielding seed, which is upon the face of all the earth, and every tree, in which is the fruit of a tree yielding seed; to you it shall be for food:" (Genesis 1:29).

YHVH didn't shame Adam and Eve into eating what was healthy. He simply provided it and called it very good. Edenic food is nourishing, colorful, satisfying, and alive. It's a gift, not a punishment.

In Edenic culture:

> Eating is an act of gratitude, not guilt.

> Boundaries are based on life and design, not deprivation.

> Nourishment is about function and connection, not thinness or trends.

Edenic eating asks: What fuels peace in my body? What honors the design? What keeps me whole, not fractured?

Idolatry of Body Image, Industry, and "Self-Care"

Modern diet culture has grown into a multibillion-dollar industry built not on truth, but on insecurity. It doesn't want you to be well—it wants you to be dependent.

It promotes:

> Body image as identity — where worth is measured in pants size or Instagram likes.

> Endless products — powders, pills, plans, and programs that promise peace but deliver pressure.

"Self-care" rituals that focus on the self rather than the soul.

Under the surface, diet culture is no different from the idols YHVH warned us about in ancient times. It demands sacrifice—your money, your mental health, your relationships, your time—and in return, it gives you temporary validation and constant striving.

> "[5] They have mouths, but they speak not;
>
> Eyes have they, but they see not;
>
> [6] They have ears, but they hear not;
>
> Noses have they, but they smell not;" (Psalm 115:5–6).

Today's idols aren't golden calves—they're curated bodies, elite wellness regimens, and "clean" lifestyles that exalt self-glory rather than Creator-designed simplicity.

Edenic living dismantles that.

It returns us to a rhythm where:

> Food supports the body without owning the mind.
>
> Health is pursued as a form of stewardship, not performance.
>
> The body is respected, not worshiped.
>
> Rest is part of the rhythm—not something to earn.

Eden Invites, Diet Culture Demands

Diet culture says: "Fix yourself."

Eden says: "Return to what you were created for."

> Diet culture says: "You're not enough."
>
> Eden says: "You are fearfully and wonderfully made—now nourish accordingly."

> Diet culture says: "Chase the image."
>
> Eden says: "Bear the image of the Creator."

When we align with Eden, we no longer eat to impress, perform, or escape. We eat to live, to worship, and to heal. And that changes everything.

III. Detoxing the Body and the Beliefs

Detox isn't just a buzzword. In the Edenic context, detox means removing what doesn't belong—not just from the body, but from the mind, emotions, and spirit. It's about letting go of what Babylon has built inside us and returning to what YHVH originally designed.

Detoxing is both physical and spiritual. You can't cleanse the body while feeding toxic beliefs. And you can't renew the spirit while clinging to substances or habits that harm the body.

Real healing requires both kinds of cleansing.

Processed Food and Pharmaceutical Dependency

Let's start with the body.

The modern food system is built on the concept of artificial abundance. Instead of real food, we are offered edible substances engineered in a laboratory to hook the brain, inflame the gut, and numb the soul.

Processed food is not just unhealthy. It is designed for addiction:

>*Sugar hijacks the brain's reward centers.

>*Refined oils inflame tissues and clog detox pathways.

>*Artificial flavors and preservatives confuse the gut microbiome.

>*Food dyes and chemical additives dysregulate hormones and behavior.

These products don't nourish. They override. They are the false prophets of nutrition. They promise pleasure, but they deliver dysfunction.

And when symptoms show up—fatigue, bloating, anxiety, skin rashes—we are taught to medicate instead of investigate. This is where the pharmaceutical cycle begins.

While emergency medicine and certain drugs are helpful in crisis, most pharmaceuticals don't heal. They manage. And often, they create new imbalances in the process. We become dependent on pills to sleep, pills to wake up, pills to cope, and pills to mask the effects of other pills.

This is not freedom.

This is Babylonian bondage dressed up as healthcare.

Eden didn't require a medicine cabinet. It required obedience, trust, and nourishment.

To return, we must ask:

What have I put into my body that YHVH never intended?

What systems have I trusted more than my Creator?

What substances am I leaning on instead of healing?

Spiritual Detox: Repentance, Renewal, Reorientation

Cleansing the body alone is not enough. Many people eat perfectly and still feel spiritually dry, emotionally stuck, or mentally anxious. That's because toxicity isn't just physical—it's spiritual.

Babylon poisons us with:

Pride disguised as "empowerment."

Fear disguised as "preparedness."

Self-worship disguised as "self-care."

Busyness disguised as "purpose."

Spiritual detox begins with one powerful word: REPENTANCE.

Not in the punishing, guilt-driven sense—but in the Hebrew sense: teshuva—to return. To reorient. To come back into alignment with YHVH.

"Create in me a clean heart, O God; And renew a right spirit within me," (Psalm 51:10).

To detox spiritually is to:

Lay down false identities.

Let go of beliefs that do not reflect the truth.

Realign with who YHVH says you are.

This is not a one-time event. It is a lifestyle of renewal. And just like physical detox, it requires rest, reflection, release, and rhythm.

Reorientation means turning away from culture and turning toward covenant. It means questioning what you've always believed about your body, your worth, your food, your habits, and replacing lies with truth.

This Is Not About Perfection. It's About Realignment.

You won't do this flawlessly. You weren't meant to.

But you were meant to live free. Free from chemicals that cloud your brain. Free from addictions that sabotage your peace. Free from shame-based thinking and performance-driven spirituality.

This detox is not punishment. It's an invitation.

It's not about discipline for its own sake. It's about clearing space for truth to flow again.

> Let go of Babylon's formulas.

> Let go of the fear of failure.

> Let go of the lie that this is too hard.

Return to the garden rhythm—where food is simple, peace is sacred, and healing comes through obedience, not effort.

IV. Returning to Simplicity and Truth

At the core of Edenic living is a simple truth: healing doesn't require complexity—it involves alignment.

The body thrives when given what it was designed to receive. The soul finds peace when it's no longer at war with itself. And the spirit reconnects when stripped of the noise and distractions that Babylon has layered over it.

But returning to simplicity takes courage. Because Babylon doesn't just complicate things—it ridicules simplicity. It glorifies the extravagant, the cutting-edge, the heavily branded, and the multi-step protocol. Simplicity, in that system, is seen as weakness or ignorance.

But Scripture tells a different story—one where simplicity becomes a form of holy resistance.

Daniel's Diet as Resistance

When Daniel and his companions were taken into Babylon, they were expected to conform. To eat the king's rich food. To abandon their identity and blend into a culture that didn't know or honor YHVH.

But Daniel knew that what he ate wasn't just physical—it was spiritual. It was about allegiance.

"But Daniel purposed in his heart that he would not defile himself with the king's dainties, nor with the wine which he drank: therefore, he requested of the prince of the eunuchs that he might not defile himself," (Daniel 1:8).

Instead, he requested only vegetables and water. Simple. Clean. Unprocessed. Plant-based.

He didn't resist with protest signs or rebellion. He resisted with a plate.

This act of dietary faithfulness wasn't just about food laws. It was a quiet stand against assimilation. It was about saying: I will not nourish myself from a system that defies the design of my Creator.

And what happened? YHVH honored his simplicity. Daniel and his friends became stronger, clearer, and wiser than the others (Daniel 1:15-17).

Their diet was their declaration.

Today, we are also surrounded by a culture that expects compliance— fast food, addictive snacks, toxic treats, indulgent holidays, and convenience disguised as care. But we don't have to submit.

When we choose Edenic food—real food—we also choose faith and freedom.

Real Food, Real Faith, Real Freedom

Real food doesn't come in boxes with nutrition buzzwords. It comes from the earth. It doesn't need a commercial to prove its benefits. It grows, it nourishes, and it testifies to the Creator's wisdom.

Real food is:

Grown, not manufactured.

Alive, not sterile.

Designed by YHVH, not branded by Babylon.

But real food isn't just about nutrients. It's about genuine faith— trusting that what YHVH provided is enough.

Faith is choosing food that heals, even when your cravings scream for comfort.

Faith is saying no to cultural pressure and yes to divine design.

Faith is believing that what the world calls "not enough" is exactly what your body was created for.

And through real food and genuine faith comes absolute freedom.

Freedom from:

> Diet culture,
>
> Food obsession,
>
> Emotional eating cycles,
>
> Industry lies,
>
> Shame and confusion.

You don't need another diet. You need a return.

Return to simplicity.

Return to what grows in the light.

Return to the rhythms that were never broken, only ignored.

Eden Isn't Complicated. Babylon Is.

YHVH's design has always been straightforward:

> Seed-bearing plants,
>
> Restful rhythms,
>
> Food prepared with love and eaten in peace,
>
> A body cared for, not punished.

This is the kind of freedom Daniel walked in.

This is the kind of clarity your body and spirit crave.

In a world full of processed noise, simplicity is prophetic. It says:

I trust my Creator more than I trust trends. I choose Eden, even in exile.

As we disentangle from the confusion of Babylon and begin returning to Edenic simplicity, it's important to clarify a vital truth:

Healing is not rebellion. Healing is restoration.

V. Proceed with Wisdom: A Note on Medication and Healing

In this chapter, we've examined the ways modern systems—especially those built on profit and performance—can distort wellness. We've challenged diet culture, called out industry-driven confusion, and questioned the over-reliance on pharmaceuticals that mask rather than mend. But none of this is an invitation to act recklessly or to make sudden, drastic changes that could endanger your health.

No one should ever stop taking prescribed medications without the guidance of a qualified medical professional.

Medications, although not the ultimate goal, often play a crucial role in stabilizing and supporting the body, especially during periods of crisis, imbalance, or transition. Many lives have been saved, and many symptoms alleviated, through compassionate and responsible medical care.

This is not about "all or nothing." This is about alignment.

You were not created to live on an ever-increasing list of prescriptions. But neither were you created to make medical decisions in isolation, out of fear, or against wise counsel. The goal is not to abruptly sever from the system, but to begin restoring what Babylon never taught us to value:

The body's God-given design to heal.

At the time of writing this book, I myself am still taking medications. Healing is not instantaneous—it is a process of returning, layer by layer, to what was always true. Five years ago, I was injecting insulin before every meal—and sometimes between meals—to manage severe blood sugar spikes. I was taking three medications for high blood pressure, along with three additional pills each day to manage blood sugar due to insulin resistance. I also relied on Zantac twice a day to manage digestive symptoms.

But then I started eating the Eden Way—real food, plant-based, unprocessed, aligned with my design. As I nourished my body and began to heal from the inside out, something remarkable happened: the need for many of those medications started to fade. Under the care of my physician, I was able to greatly reduce the medications I was taking.

Today, I take just one blood pressure pill daily and one diabetes injection weekly—and I fully believe I will be able to step away from those too, in time. Why? *Because healing takes time.* It's not a crash, a cleanse, or a moment. It's a journey of alignment, repair, and trust.

If you are starting to follow the Eden Way and are currently taking medications—especially for high blood pressure or diabetes—it's essential to inform your doctor right away. Many people experience rapid improvements in these markers within just a few weeks. Without close monitoring, continuing at the same dosage could lead to blood pressure or blood sugar dropping too low, which can be dangerous.

If these are areas of concern for you, it's also wise to monitor your own numbers at home. A simple blood pressure cuff and a reliable glucometer can provide valuable daily insights. Additionally, consider asking your doctor to check your Hemoglobin A1C and a lipid panel— as many people see remarkable improvements in these markers as the body begins to heal through proper nourishment.

So, if you're still taking medications, there is no shame here. There is no condemnation—only invitation. Invitation to begin discovering the root causes. Invitation to partner with your body rather than suppress its signals. Invitation to move forward, step by step, in the direction of freedom.

Seek root causes.

Rebuild your foundation.

Then walk forward with both discernment and peace.

Let healing be a journey, not a performance.

Let your body become trustworthy again, through how you nourish it.

Let your Creator guide your steps—and consult with your medical team—especially when and how to reduce your dependency on medications, if that time comes.

This is not about blame.

This is not about shame.

This is about awakening.

Awakening to the truth that the body is not broken by default.

Awakening to the reality that Babylon profits from your pain, but YHVH invites your restoration.

Choose that path wisely.

Walk it humbly.

And never walk it alone.

6—The Mind of Messiah: Breaking Mental Strongholds

I. Renewal as Transformation

The battle for healing doesn't begin in the stomach, the skin, or even the heart. It begins in the mind.

Before a person chooses what to eat, how to react, or whether to rest, they first process through belief. That belief may be truth… or it may be a lie wrapped in habit, fear, trauma, or pride. These entrenched beliefs—especially the ones we don't even realize we're carrying—are what Scripture refers to as strongholds.

They aren't physical walls.

They're mental and emotional fortresses—fortified places in the mind where wrong ideas have taken root and now resist truth.

What Is a Stronghold?

A stronghold, in ancient warfare, was a high, fortified structure designed to resist attack. In spiritual and emotional life, it represents a belief system or mental pattern that has been reinforced over time, often through repetition, pain, or generational programming.

Examples of strongholds include:

> "I'm not worthy of healing."

> "This is just who I am."

> "I can't change."

> "If I don't control everything, I'll fall apart."

> "I have to perform to be loved."

These aren't casual thoughts. They are lodged deep, and they shape how we eat, respond to stress, treat others, view our bodies, and relate to the Creator.

Strongholds are built when thoughts go unchallenged long enough to feel like truth.

The Mind of Messiah: What It Means to Renew

To walk in the mind of the messiah is to think as he thought, through the lens of truth, obedience, compassion, humility, and clarity. It means removing not just toxic behaviors, but the poisonous beliefs underneath them.

Yeshua constantly addressed mindsets. He taught that repentance wasn't just about outward behavior but about changing the inner perspective:

"… Repent ye; for the kingdom of heaven is at hand," (Matthew 4:17).

The Hebrew word for repent, teshuva, means return. Not merely turning from sin, but turning back to alignment: in truth, in design, in the Creator's intention.

Yeshua's entire ministry was filled with this reorientation:

> He challenged false identities
>
>> "You are not what the world calls you,"
>
>> (paraphrase of Yeshua's entire ministry).
>
> He corrected fear-based thinking
>
>> "Do not worry about tomorrow,"
>
>> (John 15:19; Matthew 5:11–12; John 17:14–16).

He revealed spiritual blindness in the religious elite and the downtrodden alike.

He spoke truth where deception had ruled, and people were set free.

To renew the mind is to reclaim territory that has been occupied by falsehood.

The Difference Between Thoughts and Truth

Not every thought is the truth.

This sounds simple, but it is revolutionary. So many people suffer—not because they are broken, but because they have believed a broken narrative for so long that it feels real.

Thought: "My body is the enemy."

Truth: "...I am fearfully and wonderfully made..." (Psalm 139:14).

Thought: "YHVH is distant and disappointed."

Truth: "Jehovah is nigh unto them that are of a broken heart, And saveth such as are of a contrite spirit," (Psalm 34:18).

Thought: "I'll never be free from this pattern."

Truth: "Then they cried unto Jehovah in their trouble, And he delivered them out of their distresses," (Psalm 107:6).

We must test every thought against the truth of Scripture and the character of YHVH. If a thought leads to fear, shame, anxiety, disconnection, or compulsion, it is likely a stronghold—not a truth.

Transformation Begins in the Mind

You can eat Edenic food, cleanse your environment, and create peaceful rhythms—but if you do it while believing you're unworthy, unloved, or powerless, your healing will stall.

Mental strongholds are like walls that block life-giving flow.

To tear them down, you must take four steps.

It begins with what is true. T.R.U.E.: Thought, Review, Unmask, and exchange.

T.R.U.E.

T – Thought: Identify the thought that entered your mind.

What are you believing?

R – Review: Compare it with the truth.

Does it align with YHVH's Word?

U – Unmask: Reject the lie.

Expose it for what it really is.

E – Exchange: Replace it with what YHVH actually says.

Speak His truth over the situation.

From distorted thoughts to divine truth—walk in what is T.R.U.E.

This is the beginning of restoration. Not with another detox, but with a renewed mind—clear, surrendered, and aligned with the mind of Messiah.

II. Emotional Sabotage Patterns

Long before you eat the wrong thing, skip the workout, explode in anger, or spiral into fatigue, a thought comes first.

That thought shapes your feelings.

Which influences your choices.

Which reinforces your beliefs.

↓

And the pattern repeats.

These are emotional sabotage patterns—internal loops that keep you stuck in cycles of fear, shame, guilt, or confusion. They don't originate from weakness or lack of willpower. They are rooted in deeper forces: unhealed trauma, embedded lies, and unseen spiritual influence.

To break them, we must first recognize them.

Negative Self-Talk: The Inner Critic Masquerading as Truth

Most people would never speak to others the way they talk to themselves.

> "I'm disgusting."

> "I always mess everything up."

> "No one cares."

> "This is just how I am—I can't change."

> "I'm too far gone to be healed."

These statements don't just reflect discouragement—they form strongholds. Over time, repeated self-talk becomes a default lens through which everything is interpreted. Even truth, when heard, is often filtered through disbelief.

Negative self-talk trains your nervous system to expect failure. It shuts down hope. It raises cortisol levels, suppresses immune function, and keeps your body locked in a state of chronic stress.

And worse, it blinds you to the truth of who you are in YHVH's design.

Shame Cycles: The Lie That You Are Your Mistakes

Shame is not the same as conviction.

> Conviction says, "You did something wrong—now come back and be restored."

> Shame says, "You are something wrong—stay hidden."

Shame is one of the most common emotional strongholds. It makes you:

> Hide your struggles,

> Perform for acceptance,

> Numb instead of feeling,

> Avoid intimacy,

> Sabotage your own progress.

What starts as a slip—a moment of weakness, overeating, losing your temper, skipping a commitment—spirals into a shame cycle. The inner voice says, See? You're a failure. You'll never change. And instead of returning to truth, you retreat deeper into the stronghold.

Shame doesn't keep you safe. It keeps you stuck.

Anxiety Loops: The Mind Racing on a Treadmill of Fear

Anxiety isn't just a mental state—it's a full-body response to perceived threat. When the mind is trained to expect danger—whether through trauma, chronic stress, or spiritual distortion—it stays on alert.

This looks like:

> Overanalyzing conversations

> Catastrophizing the future

> Obsessive planning or list-making

> Panic when plans change

> Physical symptoms like a racing heart, a tight chest, and fatigue

What fuels these loops isn't always logic—it's underlying beliefs like:

> "If I let go, something terrible will happen."

> "I must control everything to feel safe."

> "If I rest, I'll fall behind."

Anxiety becomes the nervous system's way of trying to stay ahead of pain. But it keeps the soul trapped in fear instead of freedom.

Root Causes: Trauma, Lies, and Spiritual Influence

Emotional sabotage doesn't form in a vacuum. It has roots—and until those roots are addressed, the patterns will persist.

Trauma

When something painful happens and the emotions go unprocessed, the brain creates shortcuts to protect you. These shortcuts become patterns: hypervigilance, distrust, numbing, over-control, or detachment. What was once a survival strategy becomes your normal.

Lies

Trauma often whispers lies:

> "You're too much."

> "You're not enough."

> "You'll be abandoned."

> "You're defective."

When those lies aren't confronted, they take root and shape behavior, even if your life circumstances have changed.

Spiritual Influence

Sometimes the thoughts and feelings that dominate us are not even our own. Scripture warns of spiritual forces that deceive, accuse, and confuse. These influences often reinforce the trauma and lies, creating strongholds that feel immovable.

Spiritual oppression often partners with emotional strongholds to keep you locked in fear, heaviness, and self-sabotage.

But here's the truth: these patterns can be broken.

Healing Begins with Awareness

You can't fix what you don't see. But once you recognize these sabotage patterns for what they are—*not identity, not destiny, not your fault*—you can begin to tear them down.

R.E.A.L.

R – Recognize: Identify the lie that's been shaping your thoughts.

E – Explore: Trace its root.

Where did it come from?

What triggered it?

A – Affirm: Name the truth.

What does YHVH say instead?

L – Live it: Speak it daily until it shapes how you live and think.

Replace lies with what's R.E.A.L.—Rooted, Empowering, Affirmed, and Lived. Replace the pattern with new rhythms grounded in grace and truth.

You were never created to live in cycles of fear, shame, and self-loathing.

You were created for shalom—wholeness in body, mind, and spirit.

III. Yeshua's Mindset

To restore the mind, we must not only tear down strongholds—we must also build something better in their place. That something is the mindset Yeshua taught and lived.

Yeshua's life was the perfect demonstration of what it means to be fully aligned with the will of YHVH. He wasn't driven by performance, fear, shame, or ego. His thoughts flowed from truth. His emotions were anchored in love. His actions revealed surrender, not striving.

To take on the "mind of Messiah" means to choose humility over pride, purpose over chaos, and peace over performance.

Humility: Letting Go of the Need to Prove

Yeshua never sought the spotlight. When miracles happened, he often told people not to speak of them. He wasn't building a brand—he was revealing the Father.

In a world obsessed with self-promotion, Yeshua practiced quiet obedience.

> He washed feet instead of demanding honor.

> He chose silence over self-defense.

> He prayed in solitude rather than for show.

> He refused to retaliate, even when insulted or betrayed.

This wasn't a weakness. It was spiritual strength rooted in identity. Yeshua had nothing to prove because he knew who he was and whose will he served.

When you walk in humility, you begin to release the internal pressure that drives anxiety, control, and perfectionism. You don't have to impress others or strive for validation. You align with the truth that *you are already chosen.*

Surrender: Aligning With the Father's Will

Yeshua's entire life was shaped by surrender. He said:

"My meat [food] is to do the will of him that sent me, and to accomplish his work." (John 4:34, emphasis added).

His nourishment wasn't just physical. It was purpose-driven. He did not live according to impulse or emotion. He lived according to his mission.

Even when he was exhausted, surrounded by need, misunderstood, or betrayed, he kept his mind aligned with the greater plan. He showed us what it looks like to yield to divine timing, instruction, and authority.

True surrender means trusting that:

> YHVH's ways are higher than ours
>
> Delay is not denial
>
> Healing may begin in hidden places
>
> Peace is possible even in pain.

Surrender is not passivity. It's power under authority. It's a quiet "yes" in the face of chaos. It's letting go of the need to control outcomes and instead walking in covenant and trusting YHVH.

Peace: A Settled Mind in an Unsettled World

Yeshua walked through storms without panic. He touched the untouchable without fear. He taught crowds and faced demons, yet he often withdrew for solitude and prayer.

His peace wasn't circumstantial. It was rooted in shalom (שָׁלוֹם)—the deep, Hebraic concept of wholeness, harmony, and restoration.

The world offers a temporary escape from stress. Yeshua offers internal peace that remains even when external circumstances shift.

When we adopt his mindset:

> We stop reacting from a place of fear.

> We start responding from faith.

> We speak life instead of rehearsing negativity.

> We quiet the storm within, even when storms rage outside.

Alignment With Truth and Purpose

Yeshua's thoughts were aligned with truth:

> Truth from Torah

> Truth from the Spirit

> Truth that sets people free.

Every word he spoke exposed lies and invited restoration.

This is the mindset we are called to imitate:

I.M.A.G.E.

Because we are made in the image of Elohim, and this is the mindset that reflects Him.

> I – Integrity: Truth over assumption.

> > Choose what's real, not what's presumed.

> M – Mission: Purpose over distraction.

Stay aligned with your purpose.

A – Acceptance: Grace over self-judgment.

Receive what YHVH freely gives.

G – Gratitude: Connection over comparison.

Celebrate others instead of competing.

E – Embodiment: Live this mindset daily to

Reflect the IMAGE of the Creator.

Let YHVH's I.M.A.G.E. be your lens.

What you reflect, you magnify.

You weren't created to think like Babylon.

You were created to think like Eden.

And Yeshua showed us the way.

IV. Warfare and Identity

There is a war for your mind—but it's not the kind you see on the news. It's invisible, internal, and relentless. This warfare doesn't use swords or guns. It uses thoughts, fears, memories, and words.

Every lie you believe about yourself, your body, your healing, or your relationship with YHVH is a fiery dart aimed at your identity. And every time you replace that lie with truth, you are stepping into spiritual authority.

Spiritual Battle in the Tanakh

The Hebrew Scriptures are filled with real battles—and also with the invisible battles of the soul. David faced Goliath with a sling, yes—but also with the unshakable identity of a shepherd boy who knew his Elohim.

When Goliath taunted Israel, it wasn't just a physical threat—it was psychological warfare: "You are weak. You are unworthy. You are defeated," (1 Samuel 17:8-10, paraphrased).

David's response wasn't bravado. It was truth anchored in covenant:

"'Thou comest to me with a sword, and with a spear, and with a javelin: but I come to thee in the name of Jehovah of hosts, the God of the armies of Israel, whom thou hast defied,'" (1 Samuel 17:45).

David fought from a place of identity. So did Moses when confronting Pharaoh. So did the prophets who stood against false altars. So did Yeshua when tempted in the wilderness.

They didn't win because they were strong. They won because they knew who they were—and whose they were.

Replacing Lies with Truth-Based Declarations

Spiritual warfare today is rarely visible. It looks like:

> "I'm not good enough," looping in your mind

> "I always fail," holding you back from change

> "I'll never be healed," draining your hope

You don't fight thoughts like that with effort. You fight them with truth spoken out loud, believed in the heart, and reinforced through repetition.

This is where declarations come in. You're not making things up. You're speaking what is already true in YHVH's Word, even if your feelings don't yet match.

Examples:

> "I am not what I've done. I am what YHVH says I am: chosen, whole, and called," (Isaiah 43:1; 1 Peter 2:9).

> "I reject the lie that my body is broken beyond repair. My body was designed for healing," (Psalm 103:2-3; Jeremiah 30:17).

> "I do not walk in fear. I walk in peace and power through obedience," (Isaiah 26:3; Deuteronomy 5:33).

> "I will not be ruled by shame. YHVH is near to the brokenhearted and sets the captives free," (Psalm 34:18; Isaiah 61).

Speak it until it becomes your inner dialogue. Write it. Pray it. Declare it over your meals, your mirror, and especially over your moments of weakness.

Journaling Stronghold Breakthroughs

Healing isn't always a lightning bolt. It's often a slow, steady breaking of chains, one lie at a time.

Journaling can help you:

W.R.I.T.E.

W – Witness your thoughts:

Identify recurring negative beliefs and patterns.

R – Root the origin:

> Trace where these thoughts came from—past experiences, voices, wounds.

I – Inspect with Scripture:

> Compare them to what YHVH's Word actually says.

T – Transform with truth:

> Craft a declaration that aligns with divine reality.

E – Evaluate the change:

> Track emotional and physical shifts as truth renews your mind.

Use your journal to W.R.I.T.E. your way toward freedom—one truth at a time.

Sample Journal Prompts:

> What thought is holding me back today?
>
> Where do I think this belief began?
>
> What does YHVH say about this in His Word?
>
> What would it look like to believe the truth instead?
>
> What small choice today can align with that truth?

Over time, you'll start to notice patterns breaking. Not because you're "trying harder," but because you're thinking differently.

That's how strongholds fall.

You Are Not a Victim in This Battle

You are not helpless.

You are not stuck.

You are not at the mercy of your past or your pain.

You are a vessel of the Ruach (YHVH's Spirit):

Designed for victory, not defeat.

Designed for clarity, not confusion.

Designed for shalom, not torment.

The more you renew your mind, the more the enemy loses ground.

Warfare is real, but so is your identity.

And once you walk in that truth, you become a threat to every lie you once believed.

7—The Emotional Body: When Feelings Become Physical

I. The Psychosomatic Connection

Most people divide health into separate categories: physical, emotional, and spiritual. But the body doesn't make such distinctions. It feels everything! Your emotions, thoughts, and beliefs don't just live in your mind. They echo through your cells, your hormones, your immune system, and your gut.

This connection between the mind and body is often referred to as psychosomatic. Psychosomatic is a word that has been misunderstood and even dismissed. But at its core, it means precisely what Edenic design reveals: your psyche (mind) and soma (body) are intertwined. They speak to each other constantly.

When emotions go unprocessed or trauma remains unresolved, the body doesn't forget. It stores the imprint—sometimes as tension, sometimes as inflammation, and often as chronic illness.

Stress, Trauma, and Chronic Inflammation

Not all stress is bad. Acute stress—like swerving to avoid a car accident—can be life-saving. But chronic stress—the kind that simmers under the surface day after day slowly rewires the brain and deregulates the immune system.

When you experience emotional pain but don't have space to process it, your body shifts into survival mode. This looks like:

> Adrenal overdrive (cortisol is constantly elevated)
>
> Digestive suppression (leading to bloating, IBS, or nausea)
>
> Sleep disruption (insomnia or shallow sleep)
>
> Hormonal imbalance (especially thyroid and reproductive hormones)
>
> Skin flare-ups (like eczema or acne)
>
> Low-grade inflammation that affects joints, energy, and mood

Over time, what began as emotional pain becomes physical symptoms. The trauma "moves in." It can become autoimmune conditions, fatigue, weight gain or loss, migraines, or mysterious pain that no doctor can explain.

The physical manifestation doesn't mean you're making it up. It means your body has absorbed the emotional load.

Nervous System Responses and Cellular Memory

The nervous system is your internal alarm system. It constantly scans your environment and your thoughts for signs of safety or danger. When you encounter a stressor, your body responds in one of four ways:

> Fight (anger, control, agitation)
>
> Flight (perfectionism, avoidance, anxiety)
>
> Freeze (numbness, exhaustion, detachment)
>
> Fawn (people-pleasing, codependency, loss of self)

These responses aren't choices. They're instinctive reactions trained by past experiences. If your body learned that being quiet keeps you safe, you may "freeze" under pressure. If conflict used to lead to pain, you may "fawn" to keep the peace.

Every time this cycle repeats, the body forms cellular memories. This means your cells begin to associate certain people, foods, smells, or thoughts with threat, even when the danger is no longer present.

For example:

> Someone who was verbally abused as a child may feel stomach cramps during conflict, even in adulthood.
>
> Someone who experienced abandonment may feel anxiety when a loved one is emotionally distant, even briefly.
>
> Someone who has lived in chaos may feel safe only when they're busy, even if rest is desperately needed.

These aren't just "in your head." They are embodied experiences—memories your nervous system still holds.

The Body Doesn't Lie—It Speaks

One of the most profound shifts in healing comes when you stop seeing your symptoms as the enemy and start seeing them as the messengers they are.

> The migraine may be asking you to rest.

> The rash may be asking you to release unprocessed emotion.

> The gut issue may be revealing what you've been trying to control.

> The fatigue may be a sign of grief or loss that has been repressed.

When YHVH created the body, He gave it signals, not just symptoms. And when we listen gently, without judgment, we can begin to decode what the body is trying to say.

You don't need to be afraid of your body's signals. You need to get curious.

II. Case Studies: When the Body Speaks

When the body speaks, it rarely uses words. Instead, it signals through rashes, pain, fatigue, inflammation, cravings, and imbalances. These are not merely physical malfunctions. They are messages, asking you to listen more deeply.

Below are real-life patterns—case studies of common conditions—that reveal how emotions, beliefs, and unhealed trauma can show up in the body.

Eczema and Emotional Triggers

Eczema is more than a skin issue. While food sensitivities, environmental toxins, and gut imbalances can all contribute, eczema often has emotional roots, especially in the nervous system.

Common emotional triggers for eczema:

> Unresolved anxiety,
>
> Perfectionism or pressure to please,
>
> Repressed anger or shame,
>
> A deep feeling of being unsafe or exposed.

In one example, a woman experienced full-body eczema flares during times of intense stress, but standard allergy testing found no consistent external cause. When she began an elimination diet and trauma-informed journaling practice, she discovered that her skin responded to emotional violation, feelings of being unheard, pressured, or physically, emotionally, mentally, or spiritually unsafe.

As she removed trigger foods and toxic thoughts, her skin began to clear, not just through topical creams, but through internal alignment and restoration.

The skin is the body's outermost boundary, and as such, it often reflects a boundary issue within.

Autoimmunity and Self-Rejection

Autoimmune diseases—where the body attacks its own tissues—are on the rise. While genetics and environmental factors definitely play a role, a deeper current runs beneath: self-rejection.

Many people with autoimmune issues have a long history of:

Harsh self-talk

Chronic people-pleasing

Feeling "too much" or "never enough"

Silencing their own needs

Internalizing blame for things that weren't their fault

In Hebraic thought, the body and soul are not enemies. They are integrated. So, when the soul begins to reject itself through negative thoughts and inner shame, the body may follow that pattern—attacking from within.

One man with Hashimoto's thyroiditis traced the onset of his symptoms to a season of spiritual and emotional disconnection, following years of suppressing his true identity to meet others' expectations. When he began to reconnect with truth and speak blessings over his body, not curses, his energy, immune markers, and mood all started to shift.

True healing often begins when we repent of how we've treated ourselves and return to the truth that we are "fearfully and wonderfully made" (Psalm 139:14).

Gut Health and Unprocessed Grief

The gut is often referred to as the "second brain," and for good reason. It contains a vast network of neurons and produces a significant amount of the body's serotonin, a key neurotransmitter involved in emotional regulation. However, more than that, the gut is sensitive to emotional weight, particularly in the context of grief.

Unprocessed grief—whether from loss, betrayal, sudden change, or spiritual disillusionment—can suppress digestion, slow motility, and disrupt microbial balance. Symptoms might include:

> Bloating after meals

> Nausea with emotional triggers

> Food intolerance flare-ups during anniversaries or stressful seasons

> Sudden changes in appetite

In one woman's story, chronic IBS became manageable only after she confronted the unresolved grief of a miscarriage she had never allowed herself to mourn. Through journaling, gentle fasting, and prayerful release, her gut began to calm, and her symptoms became more responsive to simple dietary changes.

The gut is more than a digestive tube. It's a feeling organ, storing the emotional residue of what we've swallowed but never digested emotionally.

Anne's Story: Hashimoto's Thyroiditis and the Edenic Diet

Anne had been battling fatigue, weight gain, brain fog, and unpredictable mood swings for years before she was finally diagnosed with Hashimoto's thyroiditis. This autoimmune disease attacks the thyroid and disrupts nearly every system in the body. Her metabolism slowed, her skin became dry and brittle, and her once-sharp memory felt like it had dulled overnight. Despite medication, her energy remained low, and flare-ups left her feeling defeated and disconnected.

Everything shifted when Anne discovered the Edenic diet—a return to the Creator's original design: whole, plant-based, and free from processed foods, animal products, and synthetic additives.

She began the journey for her thyroid health, but soon realized something deeper was happening. As she eliminated dairy, gluten, and meat, her body began to stabilize. The brain fog started to lift. Her digestion improved. She no longer needed three naps a day just to function. Her body wasn't just surviving—it was beginning to heal.

But the real breakthrough went beyond her symptoms. Anne shared, "It felt like I was waking up—spiritually and mentally. I wasn't just clearer in my thoughts; I was reconnecting with YHVH in a way I hadn't felt in years."

Her lab work confirmed what she already knew in her spirit—her thyroid antibodies had significantly decreased, and her need for medication began to taper under medical guidance. Her flares were no longer ruling her life.

Anne's journey is a living testimony: when we nourish the body in alignment with the Creator's design, healing is not only possible—it becomes inevitable.

The Edenic diet isn't a trend. It's a return to the way we were meant to live—in harmony with creation, with our purpose, and with the One who created both.

The Body as Prophet, Not Enemy

These cases aren't isolated. They are echoes of Eden lost—reminders that the body was designed to live in peace, and cannot thrive under constant emotional war.

If you're dealing with chronic symptoms, don't just ask "What's wrong with me?"

Ask, "What is my body trying to say?"

Sometimes healing begins not with another supplement or elimination of food, but with truth, compassion, and the courage to feel what you've been avoiding.

III. Inner Healing for Outer Restoration

True healing is never just skin-deep. It is layered, tender, and often invisible at first. While diet, rest, and movement are vital, emotional and spiritual healing are often the missing pieces in a person's physical recovery.

You can eat Edenic food and still carry unresolved bitterness. You can take supplements and still silently grieve losses you were never allowed to name. You can exercise and still live under the weight of shame, fear, and guilt.

The body holds on to what the heart won't release.

That's why inner healing is essential for outer restoration.

Forgiveness: Releasing What Was Never Yours to Carry

Many chronic conditions are worsened—not caused, but deepened—by resentment and emotional entanglement. This doesn't mean you've imagined your illness. It means your nervous system is carrying burdens it was never meant to bear.

Forgiveness isn't about excusing wrong behavior or pretending something didn't hurt. It's about cutting the cord that ties you to that pain, so your body can exhale.

Some signs you may need to forgive:

> Recurring mental replay of painful moments

Muscle tension, grinding teeth, clenched jaw

Spikes of pain or inflammation after emotional triggers

Struggling to rest or trust—even in safe places

Forgiveness frees your biology. It shifts your nervous system from vigilance to peace, from stress to shalom.

Repentance: Returning to Truth and Alignment

Repentance is more than saying "I'm sorry." It's a turning—a reorientation of your thoughts, choices, and direction.

Sometimes the strongest strongholds in our health come from agreements we've made with lies:

"I'll always be sick."

"I deserve this pain."

"I'm too broken to change."

Repentance involves recognizing where those lies have taken root, renouncing them, and returning to the truth of YHVH's design:

You were created to heal.

You are fearfully and wonderfully made.

You are not beyond restoration.

Repentance is powerful because it doesn't just heal the heart. It releases the body from the scripts it has been obeying.

Grief Work: Making Space for What Was Lost

Grief is not always about death. It can be about:

> A childhood you didn't have,

> A dream that never materialized,

> A body that hasn't yet healed,

> A relationship that harmed more than it helped.

Grief stored is grief multiplied. It seeps into tissues, affects sleep patterns, influences eating habits, and impacts hormones.

Doing grief work doesn't mean wallowing in sadness. It means creating space for sacred mourning—acknowledging the loss, expressing the ache, and inviting YHVH into the void.

This work can look like:

> Crying without shame,

> Writing letters to your younger self,

> Speaking aloud what was never validated,

> Praying honestly, even with questions,

> Letting yourself feel, without rushing to fix.

Grief, when held in the arms of YHVH, becomes fertile ground for compassion, maturity, and even healing.

Psalm 139: YHVH Knows Every Part

¹³ For thou didst form my inward parts: Thou didst cover me in my

mother's womb. [14] I will give thanks unto thee; for I am fearfully and wonderfully made: Wonderful are thy works; And that my soul knoweth right well.[15] My frame was not hidden from thee, When I was made in secret, and curiously wrought in the lowest parts of the earth. [16] Thine eyes did see mine unformed substance; And in thy book they were all written, Even the days that were ordained for me, when as yet there was none of them," (Psalm 139:13-16).

YHVH doesn't just know your body. He knows every layer of your inner being: your grief, your memories, your hidden wounds. Nothing is too dark or tangled for Him to unravel.

He doesn't shame your pain. He invites you to bring it to Him.

The same hands that formed you in the womb can restore you now.

IV. Tools for Healing the Emotional Body

Healing the emotional body requires more than good intentions. It calls for practical tools—simple, sacred practices that invite the nervous system to settle, the heart to open, and the body to trust again.

These tools don't erase pain, but they help repattern the body's response to it. They turn chaos into curiosity, resistance into release, and fear into a pathway for healing.

Breathwork: Resetting the Nervous System

Breath is sacred. In Hebrew, the word ruach means both "breath" and "spirit." Breath was the very substance YHVH used to animate the first human. It is still the quickest way to calm the body.

Shallow, rapid breathing keeps us in a state of fight-or-flight mode.

Deep, intentional breathing tells the body, 'You are safe now.'

Try this simple Edenic breath practice:

> Inhale through your nose for 4 counts
>
> Hold for 4 counts
>
> Exhale through your mouth for 6 counts
>
> Repeat for 2–3 minutes, focusing on peace

This isn't just relaxation. It's rewiring. Breathing out slower than you breathe in activates the parasympathetic nervous system (rest and repair) and reduces inflammation on a cellular level.

Do this before meals, during moments of stress, or before sleep to support both emotional and physical healing.

Journaling: Releasing What the Body Carries

When thoughts stay in your head, they tangle. When you write them down, you clear the clutter and make space for truth.

Journaling isn't just reflection—it's revelation. When you allow yourself to go D.E.E.P., you create space for healing, honesty, and divine presence to meet you in the hidden places.

D.E.E.P.

D – Discover triggers:

> Identify hidden emotional reactions beneath the surface.

E – Examine thought loops:

> Recognize patterns that keep you stuck.

E – Explore connections:

> Trace physical symptoms back to emotional and spiritual roots.

P – Process with Presence:

> Invite YHVH into your raw, real story for healing and transformation.

Go D.E.E.P. in your journal, because healing begins when you stop hiding.

Use prompts like:

> What emotion am I feeling right now, and where do I feel it in my body?

> What lies have I believed that need to be released?

> What is YHVH inviting me to see or surrender today?

> What boundaries do I need to honor to protect my peace?

This practice is a sacred dialogue between you, your body, and the Creator who knows your inmost parts (Psalm 139:13).

Safe Boundaries: Honoring the Body's Yes and No

Many emotional symptoms arise not from what we feel, but from feeling things we can't express or carrying burdens that aren't ours to hold.

Boundaries are not walls—they are fences with gates. They keep love in and harm out. They teach others how to treat us, and they teach us to honor the sacredness of our bodies and minds.

Safe boundaries may include:

Saying no without apology,

Stepping away from toxic conversations or relationships,

Limiting social media that fuels shame or comparison,

Carving out quiet time without guilt,

Refusing to rescue or fix others at the expense of your health.

Each time you honor a boundary, you affirm: "My peace matters. My healing matters. I am no longer available for emotional violation."

Emotions as Messengers, Not Enemies

Sadness, anger, fear, and grief are not threats—they are signals. They speak a language the body understands, often before we do.

Instead of suppressing emotions, we must learn to listen with compassion:

Sadness may be asking for rest or release.

Anger may be revealing a boundary violation.

Anxiety may be signaling an unmet need for safety.

Grief may be inviting us to slow down and honor what's been lost.

Your emotions are not sins or signs of weakness. They are sacred data.

When you stop fighting them, you can begin to partner with them in the healing process. This is how Eden is restored: one breath, one truth, one honest feeling at a time.

8—The Sabbath Rhythm of Healing

I. The Pattern from the Beginning

From the very first week of creation, YHVH established a rhythm: six days of labor, one day of rest. This was not a suggestion for tired humans. It was a divine pattern, modeled by the Creator Himself. Before sin entered the world, before there was toil, before disease, there was Sabbath (שַׁבָּת – Shabbat).

"² And on the seventh day God finished his work which he had made; and he rested on the seventh day from all his work which he had made. ³ And God blessed the seventh day, and hallowed it; because that in it he rested from all his work which God had created and made," (Genesis 2:2-30.

In Hebrew, the word for rest—Shabbat—means more than just ceasing activity. It means to return, to pause, to delight, and to restore. Sabbath is not laziness. It is a sacred alignment.

YHVH didn't rest because He was tired. He rested to establish a rhythm of renewal, a weekly return to presence, peace, and purpose.

Rest as a Sacred Rhythm

Sabbath rest was the first thing declared holy (קָדוֹשׁ, – kadosh, which means set apart) in Scripture—not a place, not a person, but time. In a world obsessed with productivity and constant movement, Sabbath is a revolutionary act of trust. It says:

> "I am not what I produce."

> "My worth is not measured by output."

> "I trust YHVH to sustain what I release."

This rhythm is not optional for those who want to live in alignment with the Edenic design. It is essential.

Exodus 20: Sabbath as Commandment and Gift

When YHVH gave the Ten Commandments, He didn't just mention the Sabbath. He expounded on it more than any other:

"[8] Remember the sabbath day, to keep it holy. [9] Six days shalt thou labor, and do all thy work; [10] but the seventh day is a sabbath [rest] unto Jehovah thy God: in it thou shalt not do any work, thou, nor thy son, nor thy daughter, thy man-servant, nor thy maid-servant, nor thy cattle, nor thy stranger that is within thy gates: [11] for in six days Jehovah made heaven and earth, the sea, and all that in them is, and rested the seventh day: wherefore Jehovah blessed the sabbath day, and hallowed it," (Exodus 20:8-11, emphasis added).

The Sabbath is a commandment, yes, but it's also a **gift**. A weekly invitation to return to Eden, to step out of Babylon's grind, and to dwell in the peace of divine presence.

Sabbath reminds the body:

> That it is not a machine.

> That rest is productive.

That healing accelerates when we stop striving.

Modern science confirms what Torah has always revealed: regular rest lowers inflammation, improves immune function, calms the nervous system, and enhances mental clarity. But long before those studies, YHVH already knew—we are rest-restored beings.

II. The Healing Science of Rest

Sabbath rest is not just a spiritual invitation. It is a physiological necessity. The human body is wired for rhythmic recovery, not nonstop performance. When we ignore the command to rest, we disrupt finely tuned hormonal cycles, overtax the nervous system, and create the biological conditions for chronic illness.

Modern science confirms what Scripture has long taught: proper rest is essential for healing.

Hormonal Reset: Cortisol, Insulin, and Sleep

The endocrine system functions on circadian and ultradian rhythms— cycles that depend on regular periods of rest, with ultradian referring to shorter biological rhythms that occur multiple times within a 24-hour day. When we break these cycles through overwork, screen exposure, stress, or disrupted sleep, we create hormonal chaos.

Cortisol, our primary stress hormone, rises naturally in the morning and falls at night. But when rest is neglected, cortisol remains elevated, leading to:

> Insomnia and fatigue,
>
> Increased inflammation,
>
> Weakened immunity,
>
> Weight gain and insulin resistance.

Studies have shown that chronic stress and insufficient rest lead to elevated cortisol and impaired insulin sensitivity, increasing the risk of type 2 diabetes and metabolic dysfunction (Liu, 2016).

Insulin, the hormone that regulates blood sugar, also depends on proper rest. Lack of sleep—even for a few nights—can impair glucose metabolism and lead to spikes in blood sugar and hunger hormones (Spiegel K., 2005).

Additionally, deep sleep is the time when the body releases growth hormone, critical for tissue repair, detoxification, and cellular renewal. Without Sabbath-style rest—including down-regulated evenings and full recovery days—this healing process is hindered.

Nervous System Regulation and Trauma Healing

The autonomic nervous system has two primary states:

> Sympathetic (fight, flight, or freeze)

> Parasympathetic (rest, digest, and heal).

Most modern people live in a state of sympathetic overdrive—constantly stimulated, triggered, and alert. But healing only happens when the parasympathetic system is dominant. Sabbath rest activates this healing state.

Practices like deep breathing, stillness, prayer, and nature immersion—all foundational to Sabbath—have been shown to:

> Lower heart rate and blood pressure,

> Reduce cortisol levels,

> Enhance emotional regulation,

> Improve trauma recovery and memory integration (Van der Kolk, 2014).

Trauma does not heal amidst hustle. It heals in safety and rhythm.

In his research on trauma and the body, Dr. Stephen Porges (2011) introduced the Polyvagal Theory, showing that healing is not just about time, but about creating rhythmic environments of safety. Sabbath is precisely that. It is a predictable, protected time where the soul can rest and the body can finally exhale.

Rest as Recovery, Not Reward

In Babylon, rest is earned after exhaustion. In Eden, rest is the foundation of life.

When we stop, we don't fall behind. We sync with our design. Hormones recalibrate. Nerves settle. The mind clears. The soul hears more clearly.

Sabbath is not a weakness. It's wisdom. It is also scientifically supported as a weekly key to sustainable healing.

III. Rhythms of Surrender

Sabbath is not just about stopping work. It is about surrendering control, stepping out of self-effort, and back into trust. In a world obsessed with productivity, independence, and optimization, rest is a radical act of faith.

Sabbath whispers:

"You are not the provider."

"You are not the sustainer."

"You are not Elohim."

While Babylon screams over.

To truly enter Sabbath, we must let go—not just of tasks, but of the illusion of control.

Letting Go of Control

Many of us keep moving not because we love our work, but because we fear what might rise in the silence:

> "If I stop, I'll fall behind."

> "If I rest, I'll lose everything."

> "If I don't hold it all together, who will?"

These thoughts are rooted in self-preservation, not divine alignment.

Sabbath breaks this cycle. It invites us to lay down the burdens of:

Constant decision-making

Emotional vigilance

Performance and perfectionism

Fixing, solving, and managing outcomes

Letting go of control doesn't mean giving up responsibility. It means releasing the outcomes and trusting that the Creator is still on the throne—even when your hands are not on the wheel.

Receiving Joy

Sabbath was never meant to be somber. It is a delight, a feast, a celebration of creation and covenant.

When we stop striving, we make space for joy to return. Not the kind manufactured through distraction or entertainment, but the kind that bubbles up from stillness, gratitude, and presence.

Joy comes in simple forms on Shabbat:

A quiet moment with tea and scripture.

Laughing with loved ones.

Lighting candles and blessing the day.

Breathing deep without rushing the next thing.

These moments are not small. They are restorative.

Stillness as Strength

Stillness is not stagnation. It is sacred grounding. In stillness, your body recalibrates, your spirit listens, and your heart remembers who you are.

"Be still, and know that I am God: I will be exalted among the nations, I will be exalted in the earth," (Psalm 46:10).

Sabbath stillness is the space where healing multiplies. When you stop, you give your nervous system permission to soften. You allow the Spirit to speak louder than your schedule. You remember that being is more valuable than doing.

Stillness is not a reward for completing your checklist. It is a birthright, built into creation itself.

Trust: The Foundation of Sabbath

Sabbath keeps us anchored in trust:

Trust that YHVH provides when we pause.

Trust that healing doesn't depend on constant striving.

Trust that you are more than your productivity.

Trust that you can lay down the heavy yoke of self-reliance.

This trust is how Eden is restored in the heart. It's not just about resting your body. It's about restoring the relationship between you and the One who called rest holy.

Sabbath isn't something we earn. It's something we receive.

It is the weekly rhythm that gently but firmly says:

"You are safe to rest. You are loved without effort. You are held."

IV. Making Sabbath Holy Again

The Sabbath was never meant to be a burdensome rule or a religious performance. It was a gift, handcrafted by the Creator as a weekly invitation to experience Eden again. To make Sabbath holy is to set it apart—not just in theory, but in action, preparation, and posture.

Many people long for the peace of Shabbat but struggle with how to practice it. In our busy, digital world, reclaiming sacred rest requires intentionality. Here's how to begin.

Sabbath Preparation: Rest Begins Before Sundown

Sabbath doesn't begin when the candles are lit. It begins in preparation.

In the Hebrew mindset, the day begins at sundown. That means Friday (Preparation Day) is a vital part of keeping Shabbat with peace, not panic. Just as manna was gathered double on the sixth day, we prepare ahead so we can truly rest.

Practical Prep Tips:

> Finish laundry, dishes, and house tidying early
>
> Make meals ahead—soups, stews, salads, or baked goods that reheat well
>
> Light candles, dim lights, and create a peaceful atmosphere
>
> Put away phones and turn off notifications
>
> Set out cozy clothes or blankets for intentional stillness

Prepare your heart: pray, journal, repent, and realign

The goal isn't perfection—it's peace.

Sabbath Foods: Nourishment Without Stress

Food is a key part of Shabbat joy—but it should never become a source of anxiety. Edenic foods—plant-based, whole, and simple—can easily be made ahead of time.

Ideas for Sabbath-Friendly Meals:

> Baked lentil loaf with roasted root veggies
>
> Oil-free vegetable soup with sourdough or spelt flatbread
>
> Chickpea salad or wrap platters
>
> Stuffed squash or sweet potatoes with herbs and tahini
>
> Fruit platters with dates and nuts for a delightfully sweet close

Make food that's nourishing and satisfying, but not labor-intensive. Let the table be about connection, not complication.

Rituals That Set the Day Apart

Shabbat becomes holy not only through what we avoid (work), but also through what we embrace. Holy habits invite the presence of YHVH into our homes and hearts.

Simple Rituals to Welcome Shabbat:

> Light two candles at sundown (symbolizing remembering and keeping the Sabbath).
>
> Bless the day aloud as a family or individually.
>
> Read Genesis 2:1–3 and a Psalm together.

Pray or sing to set your heart in alignment.

Shower or bathe as a symbolic cleansing of the week.

Journal or speak a declaration: "This is sacred time. I am resting in YHVH."

Meet with others who are members of the Yachad—a community walking in unity, healing, and truth to discuss and study the Torah (Instructions).

These rituals don't have to be rigid or ceremonial. Let them be meaningful and restful, allowing your attention to return to the Creator.

Heart Postures: Resting in Trust

More important than anything you do on Shabbat is the spirit in which you do it. Keeping the Sabbath holy means resting *with* YHVH, not merely resting *from* labor.

Check your heart:

Are you anxious or present?

Are you striving or surrendering?

Are you numbing or communing?

Shabbat invites us to:

Let go of tasks

Be present with loved ones

Dwell in gratitude

Reflect on the goodness of the Creator

Reflect on the goodness of His creation

Realign with truth, purpose, and peace

When we keep the Sabbath with intentionality, Eden becomes more than a memory—it becomes a living rhythm in our homes and hearts.

*See the Eden Way Tookbox at the end of the book for a sweet little Sabbath Poem: "Shabbat is Here!"

9—Living Water & Living Words

I. Water as a Physical and Spiritual Symbol

From the first verses of Scripture to the final scenes of restoration, water flows as a sacred symbol—one of purity, power, life, and transformation. It is no coincidence that our physical bodies are composed of over 70% water, nor that every culture and faith tradition views water as a threshold between the ordinary and the sacred.

In both creation and restoration, water holds a central place in YHVH's design.

Water at the Beginning

In Genesis 1:2, before light, land, or life, "the Spirit of God moved upon the face of the waters." Water is the first element present in creation. It is fluid, unshaped, teeming with potential. Before any order was spoken, water was there, waiting.

It was also in the Garden, flowing from four riverheads that provided nourishment and defined the boundaries of Eden (Genesis 2:10-14). The image of water was built into the blueprint of abundance.

Water in the Womb

From creation to conception, water is life's first environment. The womb—our first home—is filled with amniotic fluid, echoing the deep waters of creation. This fluid protects, cushions, and provides essential nutrients for growth.

Just as YHVH formed the earth out of the deep, He forms us in water—intimately, intentionally, and miraculously.

Water is not just symbolic. It is the substance of life and birth, spiritually and biologically.

Mikveh: Immersion and Renewal

In Hebraic practice, water is central to purification and restoration. The mikveh—a pool used for ritual immersion—symbolizes death to impurity and rebirth into a state of cleanliness and covenant. It was used for spiritual preparation, healing from illness, and returning to the community.

When John the Immerser called people to repentance in the Jordan River, he was calling them to mikveh—a turning, a washing, a new beginning. Yeshua himself was immersed in those same waters, marking the beginning of his public ministry.

Mikveh is more than tradition. It is a physical act with spiritual consequences—a reminder that YHVH heals both the seen and the unseen.

Yeshua and Living Water

Yeshua often spoke of living water—not stagnant or ceremonial, but flowing, refreshing, and life-giving. In John 7:37-38, he declared, "[37]...'If any man thirst, let him come unto me and drink. [38] He that believeth on me, as the scripture hath said, from within him shall flow rivers of living water.'"

This imagery links the physical thirst of the body with the spiritual thirst of the soul. His teachings offered a kind of water that reached deeper than the tongue—one that healed identity, washed shame, and rehydrated the spirit.

Hydration and Cellular Healing

Science supports what Scripture has long symbolized—water is vital for healing. Every system in the body relies on adequate hydration:

Digestion

Detoxification

Nutrient dispersion

Joint lubrication

Temperature regulation

Cognitive clarity

Emotional regulation

Cellular communication

Immune defense

Even mild dehydration increases cortisol (the stress hormone), reduces energy, and slows healing processes. Chronic dehydration has been linked to headaches, brain fog, joint pain, and increased inflammation (Popkin, 2010).

Hydrating with pure, mineral-rich water is one of the simplest and most Edenic practices you can reclaim.

Restoring the Waters Within

Water is never just about quenching thirst. It is about alignment with flow. It's about returning to the design where water:

> Was present before time

> Delivered us into the world

> Continues to wash, nourish, and renew

Let every glass of water you drink become a moment of return—a sacred sip, a whispered reminder:

> "I am made to flow. I am made to heal. I am made to carry living water."

II. The Power of Speech

Words are not neutral. In Scripture, they are never just sounds—they are agents of life or death. In the beginning, YHVH spoke creation into existence. The earth was shaped not by tools, but by words. And just as His words carried the power to form galaxies, our words have the power to build or break, to bless or burden.

"Death and life are in the power of the tongue; And they that love it shall eat the fruit thereof," (Proverbs 18:21).

Every time we speak, we plant something. And eventually, we eat the fruit of what we've said—whether that's peace or anxiety, courage or condemnation, alignment or disconnection.

Self-Talk: When You Preach to Yourself

We are always listening to ourselves, whether we realize it or not. The internal monologue you carry becomes the script that shapes your life.

If your self-talk sounds like:

> "I'll never be well."

> "My body is broken."

> "I'm too far gone."

Then your nervous system hears that, your beliefs begin to agree with it, and your body responds accordingly.

But if you begin to say:

> "My body is healing."

> "I am made in the image of Elohim."

> "Each day I align more with wholeness."

Then you begin to shift your inner atmosphere—spiritually, emotionally, and physically.

Science confirms that self-affirming language can rewire neural pathways, reduce stress, and improve problem-solving and resilience (Creswell, 2005). Your words teach your brain how to think, and your body how to respond.

Prayer: Language of Intimacy and Authority

Prayer isn't a formula—it's a dialogue of trust. When we pray, we are not just asking—we are also aligning. Prayer realigns our thoughts, emotions, and expectations with YHVH's will and character.

The Hebrew prayers of Scripture—such as the Shema (Deuteronomy 6:4-9) are not casual. They are covenant declarations, meant to be spoken daily, aloud, and with heart.

Prayer is also where truth confronts lies:

> "Abba, I feel abandoned... but You say You will never leave me."

> "I feel weak... but You are my strength."

> "This symptom scares me... but You are the Healer."

Spoken prayer invites the living presence of Elohim into the moment—and into the cells of our bodies. It is not passive. It is restorative warfare.

Declarations: Speaking Life on Purpose

Declarations are proactive truth-statements grounded in YHVH's character and promises. They are not wishful thinking. They are tools to break agreement with lies and anchor ourselves in reality, even when we don't feel it yet.

Examples of Edenic declarations:

> "I choose life today in my thoughts, choices, and actions."

> "My body was designed for healing, and I align with

that design."

"I am not a victim. I walk in authority, peace, and purpose."

"I break agreement with the lie that I am too far gone. I receive truth and wholeness."

Declarations may feel awkward at first, but as you persist, your body and spirit begin to recognize the sound of truth.

Your Voice Restores Atmospheres

You carry power in your mouth—enough to shift an environment, calm a storm of anxiety, bless your food, or speak healing over your own nervous system. This is not New Age. It is Edenic.

In Genesis, the serpent used words to deceive. But YHVH gives you words to deliver.

So, speak:

Life over your health.

Peace over your home.

Truth over your identity.

Restoration over your relationships.

Let your tongue return to its Edenic purpose: to create, not destroy—to bless, not curse—to align, not distort.

III. YHVH's Name and Healing Authority

There is power in a name. But when it comes to the Name of the Creator, that power is not merely symbolic—it is restorative, sacred, and embodied. In a world that substitutes titles for identity and vague references for relationship, the Name YHVH (יהוה) remains a vital key to spiritual and even physical healing.

The Tetragrammaton: Breath, Being, and Frequency

The Name YHVH is made up of four Hebrew letters—Yod, Heh, Vav, Heh—referred to as the Tetragrammaton. Unlike names given by man, this Name was revealed by Elohim Himself. In Exodus 3:15, YHVH says:

"...this is my name for ever, and this is my memorial unto all generations."

Some modern scholars and teachers suggest that the Name YHVH may echo the very sound of breath—inhale Yah, exhale Veh—reminding us that the divine is present in every breath we take. While not directly recorded in ancient texts, the reverence for the Name as "unutterable" aligns with its sacred rhythm (Rohr, 2014).

Try it: Yod... (inhale)

               Heh... (exhale)

               Vav... (inhale)

               Heh... (exhale)

The Name becomes not just something we speak—but something we breathe. Every human, from birth to death, echoes His Name with every breath.

This rhythm of the Name is also understood to carry a resonant frequency. Sound therapy and frequency research now confirm what the ancients perceived: certain tones bring healing, peace, and cellular alignment (Bartel, 2013). If creation was spoken into existence by the voice of Elohim, it follows that His Name carries restorative resonance as well.

Titles vs. the True Name

Over time, the sacred Name was replaced with titles: Lord, God, Adonai. While these titles may carry reverence, they are not personal identifiers. They describe a role, not a relationship.

Substituting the Name with titles:

> Diminishes the intimacy of calling on the One who named Himself

> Erases the Hebraic identity of the Creator

> Dilutes the authority and distinctiveness of His revealed character.

Yeshua did not come declaring "the Lord," but making the Father, YHVH, known (John 17:6). He used and taught the Name. When we use it, we step into that exact alignment. Not superstition, but obedience. Not legalism, but legacy.

Healing and the Name

Scripture shows again and again that healing is tied to the Name of YHVH:

"…I am Jehovah that healeth thee," (Exodus 15:26).

"The name of Jehovah is a strong tower; The righteous runneth into it, and is safe," (Proverbs 18:10).

"…whosoever shall call on the name of Jehovah shall be delivered," (Joel 2:32).

When we pray, declare, or sing the proper Name, we align ourselves with covenantal authority. We return to Edenic identity, where the Creator walked with His creation by Name, not title.

Speaking the Name with Reverence and Boldness

Reclaiming the Name is not about correcting others. It's about restoring the relationship. We speak it not for performance, but for presence. We honor it not out of fear, but because it is sacred, healing, and true.

Let your mouth become a vessel of alignment where speech, breath, and spirit all echo one cry:

> "YHVH, you are my Source. I remember who You are,
>
> and who I am in You."

IV. Words That Heal

Words can bruise, and words can bind. But words can also bless, rebuild, and restore. Scripture, science, and lived experience all testify to the power of speech, not just to describe reality, but to shape it. When we begin speaking life over our bodies and truth into our pain, we align with the Creator's intent: to heal with our mouths as well as our hands.

Blessing the Body

In many spiritual traditions—especially Hebraic ones—blessing isn't a passive wish. It's a spoken activation of truth. To bless is to call forth what is good, to name what is sacred, and to speak destiny into being.

Our bodies, worn by stress, trauma, and culture's shame-based messages, long to be blessed again, not scrutinized and not punished. Blessed.

Try this:

"I bless my nervous system with peace."

"I bless my gut with gentleness and nourishment."

"I bless my skin with renewal and protection."

"I bless my hormones with balance and harmony."

"I bless my lungs with every breath of YHVH's Name."

When we speak blessings, we retrain our inner dialogue to echo Eden. We remind the body that it is not a battlefield, but a temple. Blessing becomes a form of worship, honoring the vessel YHVH handcrafted with love and wisdom.

Speaking Truth to Trauma

Trauma often embeds lies deep into the body's memory:

"You're not safe."

"You deserved it."

"You're broken forever."

"You'll never heal."

These are not just thoughts. They become internal scripts that shape physiology, behavior, and belief.

But truth spoken aloud can unravel those lies.

Words that heal trauma don't deny pain. They interrupt it with reality:

> "What happened to me was not my fault."

> "I am not what they did to me."

> "I am healing, even when it's slow."

> "YHVH sees me, knows me, and walks with me."

> "I am safe now. My body can rest."

Trauma may begin in silence, but healing often begins with a voice— your voice.

When you speak healing words, you create a new pattern in your nervous system. You activate hope. You remind every cell that it is safe to stop bracing and start rebuilding.

The Word Made Flesh

In the beginning, the Word of YHVH created. Today, your words still create.

You can speak to your body and your past the way YHVH spoke to chaos:

> **"Let there be light," (Genesis 1:3).**

> Light in your mind.

> Light in your cells.

Light in your memories.

Speak life.

Speak blessings.

Speak the truth.

And watch what begins to heal.

10—From Surviving to Sovereignty

I. The Shift from Victim to Steward

We were not created to merely survive. We were designed to steward, reign, and create, in partnership with our Creator. The Edenic mandate in Genesis 1:28 is clear:

"…'Be fruitful, and multiply, and replenish the earth, and subdue it; and have dominion over the fish of the sea, and over the birds of the heavens, and over every living thing that moveth upon the earth.'"

This wasn't a call to dominate in fear or force. It was a call to responsible sovereignty, to care for creation, starting with ourselves. But trauma, disconnection, and cultural programming often push us into victimhood, where we live reactively instead of intentionally.

From Survival Mode to Kingdom Mode

Survival mode is understandable in times of crisis, but it was never meant to be permanent. Signs of survival mode include:

Constant fatigue or burnout

Fear-based decision-making

Numbing behaviors (overeating, scrolling, overworking)

Apathy and self-neglect

Waiting for rescue instead of taking action

YHVH didn't create us to be helpless. He made us in His image—with creativity, choice, and courage. Stewardship is how we return to that image.

Taking Dominion Starts with You

Before we take dominion over land, finances, or time, we must first take dominion over our inner terrain:

Thoughts

Emotions

Habits

Beliefs

Health

This doesn't mean self-will or perfection. It means partnership—co-laboring with YHVH's Spirit to restore order where there has been chaos.

You begin to say:

"I may not control everything that happened to me…

But I choose how I respond now."

"I am not what I've endured…

I am who I decide to become in YHVH."

"My body, mind, and choices

Are under my stewardship, not my shame."

This is the first step from surviving to sovereign living: choosing to engage rather than disengage.

Breaking Passive Patterns

Victimhood often comes with passivity. It sounds like:

"This is just how I am."

"Nothing ever works for me."

"They always ruin my progress."

"Why even try?"

But YHVH's call to dominion is active. It's not waiting for the perfect conditions. It's planting in famine, rebuilding in ruins, and reclaiming what was lost.

To break passive patterns, you must:

1. Identify self-sabotaging scripts

2. Repent of agreement with lies and labels

3. Speak truth-based declarations daily

4. Take consistent, small actions that reinforce sovereignty

5. Surround yourself with people and practices that call you higher

You were not designed to be a powerless bystander in your own life. You were created to govern your space with wisdom and shalom.

II. Sovereignty Over the Flesh

Sovereignty isn't just a spiritual principle—it's a lifestyle of embodied obedience. In Eden, the body was in perfect submission to the spirit. There was no war between craving and calling, between hunger and holiness. But once disobedience entered the garden, the flesh began demanding what the spirit used to govern.

To return to Edenic living, we must reclaim sovereignty over the flesh, not through shame or punishment, but through Spirit-led discipline.

Choosing Obedience Over Craving

Cravings aren't always physical. Sometimes they're emotional, trauma-driven, or culturally conditioned. We crave sugar when we're exhausted. We crave escape when we're overwhelmed. We crave control when we feel insecure.

But cravings, when left unchecked, become masters, not messengers. And we were never meant to be enslaved by our appetites.

"...I have set before thee life and death, the blessing and the curse: therefore, choose life, that thou mayest live, thou and thy seed;" (Deuteronomy 30:19).

Obedience is a form of sovereignty. When we choose what nourishes instead of what numbs, we return to the pattern of Eden, where the fruit we eat is in harmony with the truth we believe.

Training the Body

The body, like a garden, must be cultivated.

>   Left alone, weeds grow.

>   Without structure, chaos returns.

Discipline is not cruelty. It is alignment: aligning our flesh with consistent training to bring it into agreement with our spirit.

This might look like:

>   Eating whole, Edenic foods when your body screams for sugar,

>   Moving your body when you'd rather stay stagnant,

>   Resting on the Sabbath when you feel driven to produce,

>   Choosing stillness over stimulus,

>   Saying "no" to what flatters your flesh but steals your peace.

We don't train the body to punish it. We train it so that it becomes a vessel of peace, not chaos.

Renewing Discipline Through Delight

The world teaches discipline as a duty. Eden teaches discipline as delight.

In Hebrew thought, the word for discipline (mûsār – מוּסָר) is closely linked to instruction and correction that guides one toward wisdom and a fulfilling life. It's not harsh. It's holy.

Instead of thinking:

> "I have to give this up,"

We begin thinking:

> "I get to align with life."

Discipline becomes less about restriction and more about freedom from compulsion.

From Flesh-Driven to Spirit-Led

Sovereignty over the flesh does not come through willpower alone. It comes through spirit partnership. As we walk in intimacy with YHVH, our desires shift. Our cravings recalibrate. Our bodies become allies in the work of healing and purpose.

You were not created to be ruled by your flesh. You were made to walk in dominion, balance, and alignment.

III. Sovereignty Over the Mind and Emotions

True sovereignty doesn't stop with the body. It must extend to the thoughts we think and the emotions we feel. The mind and emotions were given to us by YHVH as part of our design. They are not enemies. But when left unguarded or unhealed, they can begin to rule us, rather than serve us.

Restoring Eden means reclaiming governance over our inner world.

Emotions as Tools, Not Tyrants

Emotions are not bad. They are signals, not verdicts—messengers, not masters. Anger may reveal injustice. Sadness may expose loss. Fear may point to vulnerability. But none of these emotions are meant to control our choices.

When we give emotions the throne, we:

> React instead of respond,
>
> Self-sabotage out of fear or shame,
>
> Avoid growth because it feels uncomfortable,
>
> Over-identify with temporary feelings.

Sovereignty over emotions means acknowledging them without bowing to them. It's learning to say:

> "I feel this, but this will not lead me."
>
> "This feeling is real, but it is not the final truth."
>
> "I honor my emotions by listening, but I rule my life by wisdom."

When our emotions are trained by truth, they become partners in healing, not barriers to it.

Setting Boundaries: Guarding the Garden Within

In Eden, YHVH placed boundaries. Certain trees were permitted; one was not. This wasn't cruelty—it was protection. Boundaries are Edenic. They say:

"This is sacred."

"This space needs protection."

"I honor myself and others by defining limits."

Emotional sovereignty requires boundaries that guard:

Your thoughts (What do I allow myself to dwell on?)

Your time (Who and what gets access to my energy?)

Your heart (Do I say yes out of peace or out of fear?)

Your healing (Am I placing myself in environments that support restoration or environments that sabotage it?)

You are not selfish for setting boundaries. You are wise.

Affirming Identity: Knowing Who You Are

You cannot walk in sovereignty if you are confused about your identity. When you don't know who you are, you become vulnerable to manipulation, fear, and false beliefs.

Affirming your identity means declaring the truth, even when your emotions haven't caught up:

"I am made in the image of Elohim."

"I am not my trauma, my diagnosis, or my past."

135

"I have authority over my thoughts and emotions."

"I am deeply loved, seen, and called to live fully."

You were never meant to live at the mercy of your moods. You were created to steward your mind and emotions with grace and clarity.

From Turmoil to Shalom

The fruit of sovereignty is shalom—a whole, unshaken, deeply anchored peace. When your inner world is ruled by truth and order, your outer world begins to reflect it.

Take back the reins. Your mind was made to think with YHVH. Your emotions are meant to flow without overwhelming you. Your heart was made to host peace.

IV. Authority in the Spirit

True sovereignty begins with stewardship of the body and mind, but it culminates in spiritual authority. We were not just created to survive hardship or manage symptoms. We are empowered to walk in spiritual authority, exercising dominion in the unseen realms just as we do in the physical.

From the garden to the wilderness, and from Torah to the teachings of Yeshua, the pattern is clear: the children of YHVH are not powerless. We are called to bind what hinders, loose what heals, and speak with Heaven's authority.

Prayers of Binding and Loosing

The Hebrew worldview understands that the physical and spiritual are intertwined. What happens in the spirit affects the body, and vice versa. That's why Yeshua taught His disciples the practice of binding and loosing (Matthew 18:18):

> "'Verily I say unto you, What things soever ye shall bind on earth shall be bound in heaven; and what things soever ye shall loose on earth shall be loosed in heaven.'"

To bind means to restrict or forbid what is unlawful or destructive— fear, lies, spiritual oppression, torment.

To loose means to release or permit what aligns with the Kingdom— healing, peace, truth, restoration.

These prayers are not magic formulas. They are acts of covenant partnership with YHVH. When prayed with discernment and faith, they become tools of liberation:

> "I bind the spirit of fear and confusion."

> "I loose the peace and clarity of the Ruach HaKodesh."

> "I bind the cycle of self-sabotage and shame."

> "I loose grace, healing, and holy discipline."

These are not empty declarations. They are spiritual legislation.

Spiritual Gifts in Healing and Restoration

YHVH gives gifts to His people not to elevate individuals, but to edify, heal, and restore. These gifts are not reserved for religious professionals. They are part of the birthright of the Body.

Some of the spiritual gifts connected to healing and restoration include:

Discernment – the ability to recognize root causes, spiritual oppression, or emotional strongholds.

Word of knowledge – insight into hidden pain or unresolved trauma.

Gift of healing – prayer, touch, or presence that initiates physical or emotional restoration.

Exhortation – speaking life and encouragement that activates growth.

Intercession – standing in the gap for someone in spiritual battle or despair.

These gifts are not performances. They are tools of Edenic restoration, meant to return us to wholeness in body, soul, and spirit.

If you are walking in obedience, intimacy, and alignment with YHVH, then you carry authority, not because of your name, but because of His Name dwelling in you.

Walking in Spiritual Dominion

To walk in spiritual authority, remember to shine your LIGHT:

L — Live from identity: Know who you are—a vessel of YHVH's Spirit, not a victim of your past.

I — Internal cleansing: Clean your spiritual house through repentance, forgiveness, and releasing bitterness.

G — Guard your words: Speak with intention, using your words to bind lies and loose truth.

H — Hope in prayer: Pray with expectancy—not begging, but

believing.

T — Take action with your gifts: Use your gifts not for fame, but for freedom—for yourself and others.

You were never meant to just cope.

You were created to reclaim, restore, and reign—in love, not fear; in power, not performance; in truth, not trauma.

This is Eden restored in spirit and sovereignty.

11—Making Your Home Eden Again

I. Your Environment Matters

In the original garden, everything was aligned—not just food and function, but atmosphere. Eden wasn't simply a place of nourishment; it was a space of peace, order, and divine presence. What surrounded Adam and Eve contributed to their well-being. Today, the same principle holds true: your physical environment can either nurture healing or hinder it.

The Space Around You Reflects the Space Within

Our homes often mirror our internal condition:

Clutter may reflect mental overwhelm.

Chaos may reflect spiritual disconnection.

Toxicity (chemical, relational, or emotional) can mirror unhealed trauma.

However, the good news is that just as trauma can shape an environment, intentional peace can also reshape it.

When you begin to restore your physical space to reflect your values—wholeness, calm, and connection—you send a message to your nervous system:

"It's safe here. You can heal here."

Healing Requires a Safe Nest

True restoration thrives in safety and stillness. Your home becomes a healing tool when it provides:

Visual peace – Clear surfaces, soft natural colors, order

Auditory calm – Gentle music, quiet space, nature sounds

Sensory nourishment – Clean air, soft fabrics, natural materials

Emotional sanctuary – Boundaries, forgiveness, joyful memories

You don't need a Pinterest-perfect home. You need a space that supports shalom—nothing missing, nothing broken.

Peace, Order, and Purity: The Edenic Blueprint

Peace is not just emotional—it's atmospheric. When you cultivate peace in your home, you make room for the presence of YHVH.

Order brings clarity. Genesis 1 shows YHVH creating through the principle of dividing and assigning. When we put things in their proper place, both physically and spiritually, we create an environment that reflects the Creator's pattern.

Purity extends beyond food or water. To create a pure environment, remember PURITY:

P — Purge toxins: Remove harmful cleaning products and synthetic fragrances.

U — Upgrade your atmosphere: Filter your water and air for cleaner living.

R — Reduce noise: Limit digital distractions and emotional clutter.

I — Inspire with words: Speak truth and blessing within your walls.

T — Tend your space: Keep your home and mind aligned with peace and order.

Y — Yield to stillness: Allow your spirit to breathe and rest in a calm environment.

Purity creates a sanctuary where your spirit can thrive.

Making Eden Tangible

You don't need to move to the country or renovate your house to begin. Eden starts with small choices:

A corner for prayer and reflection,

Removing harsh lighting or loud media,

Playing Scripture or instrumental worship,

Diffusing essential oils instead of chemical sprays,

Displaying reminders of your identity and truth.

When you reclaim your home as sacred space, it becomes more than shelter. It becomes a sanctuary.

II. Detoxing the Home

When we think of detox, we often think of juice cleanses or supplements. However, true healing also requires us to detoxify our living spaces, especially the areas where we eat, sleep, bathe, and breathe. Your home environment can either contribute to inflammation or help your body and spirit thrive.

Eden was a toxin-free zone. No synthetic chemicals. No hormone disruptors. No air fresheners that were made in laboratories. It was pure. And while we can't return to that exact state, we can honor the pattern by creating a home that nourishes and protects.

*See The Eden Way Toolbox at the back of the book for a full checklist.

The Hidden Toxins in Your Home

Many modern homes are saturated with toxins disguised as "normal." Common culprits include:

Plastics: Found in food storage containers, water bottles, and kitchen tools. Many contain BPA, phthalates, and other endocrine disruptors that can interfere with hormone function, weight regulation, and immune system function.

Fragrance: Air fresheners, scented candles, laundry detergent, and cleaning products often contain synthetic chemicals that are linked to asthma, migraines, skin irritation, and hormonal disruption.

Conventional cleaners: Bleach-based and ammonia-heavy products may kill germs, but they also expose your lungs, skin, and endocrine system to harsh compounds.

Nonstick cookware: Teflon and similar coatings release toxic fumes when heated, and they break down over time causing these toxic compounds to leach into food.

Personal care items: Lotions, shampoos, toothpaste, and makeup often contain parabens, sulfates, dyes, and preservatives that your skin absorbs directly into the bloodstream.

These exposures can contribute to low-grade inflammation, autoimmune flares, mood disturbances, hormonal imbalance, and more.

*See The Eden Way Toolbox at the back of the book for a full checklist.

Creating a Low-Inflammation Kitchen

Your kitchen is the heart of your home—and the starting point of your health journey. To restore Eden here:

Replace plastics with:

> Glass jars, stainless steel containers, beeswax wraps
>
> Silicone lids and baking mats (food-safe and reusable)

Ditch processed ingredients for:

> Whole food staples in bulk jars
>
> Organic spices, herbs, and real salt
>
> Fresh produce washed and ready to use

Swap cookware and tools:

> Cast iron, stainless steel, or ceramic cookware
>
> Bamboo or stainless utensils
>
> Avoid scratched nonstick pans and plastic spatulas

Purify your water:

> Invest in a quality water filter (such as Pure One or AquaTru)
>
> Store drinking water in glass containers, not gallon jugs of plastic

Clean with conscience:

> Vinegar, baking soda, essential oils, and castile soap make powerful, safe cleaners
>
> Diffuse oils like lemon, tea tree, or lavender instead of using aerosol sprays

145

*See The Eden Way Toolbox at the back of the book for a full checklist.

Detoxing the Bathroom and Laundry Space

In the bathroom:

> Choose fragrance-free or essential oil-scented soaps and shampoos

> Use mineral-based deodorants instead of antiperspirants with aluminum

> Ditch plastic toothbrushes for bamboo options

> Swap store-bought lotions for tallow balm or shea butter blends

In the laundry room:

> Replace detergent pods and dryer sheets with fragrance-free, non-toxic alternatives like soap nuts or mineral-based powders,

> Use wool dryer balls with a few drops of essential oil

> Skip fabric softeners and static sprays—they coat clothes in chemicals

*See The Eden Way Toolbox at the back of the book for a full checklist.

Making the Shift Sustainable

You don't have to do it all at once. Detoxing your home is a process of alignment, not perfection. Start with what touches your skin, enters your food, or fills your lungs. As each item runs out, replace it with something better. A cleaner, calmer home doesn't just support your body; it invites the Ruach (YHVH's Spirit) to dwell in purity and peace.

III Where Healing Lives: The Power of Sacred Space

Your home doesn't need cathedral ceilings or stained-glass windows to be holy ground. In the Edenic model, sanctuary is not about grandeur. It's about presence. Eden was not only a garden of provision, but a place of divine connection, order, and rest. You don't need to move to a mountain or retreat to a monastery to experience this. You can begin by turning your own home into a micro-Eden—a sacred space for wholeness.

When you intentionally shape your home's atmosphere, you don't just create a pleasing environment. You invite healing. You begin to reestablish the Edenic flow where your body, mind, and spirit find rhythm and rest.

What Makes a Space Sacred?

A sanctuary isn't defined by expensive furnishings or perfect minimalism. It's formed by what you allow to dwell there. To make your home a place of restoration:

> Create space for worship — a chair, a journal, a candle, or even a window seat can become a prayer altar.
>
> Welcome the Spirit aloud — "YHVH's Ruach, you are welcome here."
>
> Establish peace — reduce clutter, play calming music, and remove any spiritual chaos, such as resentment or unspoken tension.

> Surround yourself with intentional objects — Scripture art, handmade crafts, family heirlooms, natural materials like wood, wool, stone, and linen. Choose items that speak life.

This is not about decorating—it's about dedicating. Every item, sound, scent, and word spoken can be part of restoring Eden in your own space.

The Sensory Anchors of Sanctuary

What we hear, see, and smell all influence our inner state. Use your senses as allies in healing:

> Music: Scripture songs, psalms, soft instrumentals—these nourish the spirit. Use them during cooking, cleaning, and the Sabbath.

> Lighting: Let sunlight in during the day; use candles or warm lighting in the evening. Avoid harsh overheads and blue light before bed.

> Aroma: Diffuse essential oils like frankincense, myrrh, or citrus. Simmer cinnamon and clove or lemon and orange peels on the stove before Sabbath. Let your home smell like rest and restoration.

When your surroundings align with peace, they send a message to your nervous system:

> "You're safe here. You can heal here."

Rhythms that Invite Shalom

Sacred homes follow sacred rhythms:

Morning peace: Start your day with gratitude and quiet, rather than the news or notifications.

Meal blessings: Even the simplest food becomes sacred when offered and consumed with gratitude.

Evening wind-down: Reduce noise. Light a candle. End the day with prayer or reflection.

Sabbath preparation: Set the tone every Friday by shifting music, food, lighting, and mood. Let Sabbath enter your home like a royal guest.

These patterns offer consistency in a chaotic world and become anchors for your family's healing.

How a Sanctuary Heals

When your home becomes a place of safety, it does more than comfort. It rewires the nervous system. It teaches your body and brain to downshift, let go, and repair.

A sanctuary provides:

Predictable rhythms that create emotional trust.

Sensory support that calms trauma response.

Emotional safety where tears, joy, silence, and laughter are welcome.

A spiritual climate that is clean, peaceful, and connected.

The result is not perfection—it's presence.

Restoring Eden Room by Room

You don't have to overhaul your whole home at once. Start with the room you spend the most time in. Light a candle. Play soft music. Remove what distracts or clutters. Add what brings peace. Let each space whisper:

"This is sacred ground."

"Here, we walk with YHVH again."

And in time, your home will not just be a shelter, but a sanctuary where healing flows like a river, and Eden begins to bloom again.

IV. Creating a Safe Place for the Soul

There is a profound difference between a house that looks beautiful and a home that feels safe. One impresses the eye, but the other ministers to the soul.

In Eden, Adam and Eve were not ashamed. They were fully known and unafraid. That kind of openness and safety doesn't come from perfect furniture placement or seasonal decorations. It comes from the presence of YHVH dwelling in a space intentionally made for Him.

Hospitality to the Ruach (Holy Spirit)

Hospitality isn't just for guests. It's a posture of welcome to the Divine. It says to the Ruach HaKodesh:

"Come rest here. Come guide here. This space is Yours."

We often invite people into our homes, but we forget to consciously invite the Spirit of YHVH.

A home that welcomes the Ruach:

> Feels peaceful even when it's quiet.
>
> Is filled with the fragrance of truth and love.
>
> Prioritizes prayer, rest, and worship.
>
> Makes room for honesty, tears, laughter, and stillness.
>
> Responds to conviction without shame.

This kind of hospitality doesn't require a specific aesthetic—it involves surrender.

Sanctuary Over Showcase

Modern culture pressures us to curate homes that perform well on camera. But an Edenic home doesn't strive to be showcased. It longs to be set apart. It is not styled for Instagram but prepared for intimacy with YHVH and connection with others.

A sanctuary home may have:

> Worn but loved furniture that's been the backdrop of prayer and healing,
>
> A kitchen full of nourishing ingredients, not spotless countertops,
>
> A living room where books, journals, and blankets are scattered like breadcrumbs leading to peace,
>
> Space for movement, rest, music, and meals that feed the body and soul,

It's a home where guests exhale and say, "I don't know why, but I feel peace here." Where they aren't in a hurry to leave.

That peace is the presence of the Creator, dwelling in a home that has been made holy by intention.

Creating That Safe Place

To build this kind of sanctuary:

1. Pray over every room. Dedicate it for its purpose—rest, nourishment, learning, worship.

2. Speak life into the walls. Declare that this is a place of peace, truth, and wholeness.

3. Remove what hinders. Whether it's spiritual clutter, toxic products, or digital chaos—simplify to sanctify.

4. Invite your family or housemates into the rhythm. A sanctuary flows best when built in unity.

5. Welcome the Ruach each day. Say it out loud if needed: "You are welcome here, Spirit of the Living God."

Your home was never meant to be a museum. It was always meant to be a meeting place between heaven and earth.

When you choose sanctuary over showcase, your home becomes not just a refuge from the world, but a holy launchpad into healing, purpose, and presence.

12—Community: Healing Beyond the Self

I. The Original Design: Made for Relationship

'"…It is not good that the man should be alone…"' (Genesis 2:18).

From the beginning, Eden was never a solo journey.

YHVH could have placed Adam in a perfect garden, given him meaningful work, and left him alone to thrive, but He didn't.

Instead, the Creator paused and declared something "not good."

"It is *not good* for man to be alone…" (Genesis 2:18).

Even in paradise, connection was still essential.

Eden Was a Fellowship

The garden was a place of communion, not just between mankind and the Creator, but between humans themselves. In Eden, Adam and Eve shared:

Conversation — honest, unfiltered, relational exchange

Co-laboring — tending the garden side-by-side

Covering — both physical and emotional safety in each other's presence

Companionship — joy in shared rest, purpose, and worship

Healing wasn't something to hide. There was no shame to mask, no masks to wear, and no wounds to compare. They were naked and unashamed—fully seen and wholly safe.

That's the blueprint of wholeness we still crave.

The Wound of Isolation

Fast forward to our modern world, and many are surrounded by people yet feel deeply alone. We scroll past hundreds of faces daily and still carry wounds no one sees. We've been conditioned to heal in silence, to endure pain, and to confuse independence with strength.

But healing doesn't thrive in isolation.

It multiplies in connection.

When someone hears your pain and says, "Me too," healing begins to expand.

When you pray together, eat together, cry together—Eden peeks through again.

When your body is tired, and someone intercedes for you, the garden grows stronger.

We were not created to walk this journey alone. Restoration is a personal journey, but it is sustained and deepened in community.

The Circle Restored

As you've walked through the pages of this book, you've reclaimed Eden in your meals, your thoughts, your emotions, your rest, and your home. Now, it's time to open the gate and invite others in.

Eden is not just where you are returning—it's a space you carry and extend. It becomes real when you:

Share your story with vulnerability,

Host others around a table of real food and real conversation,

Pray with and for someone who is weary,

Create space in your home where shame can't stay,

Say "yes" to showing up, again and again, even when it's hard.

Healing accelerates when we are seen, supported, and sent.

From Me to We

You are not just a receiver of Eden.

You are now a releaser of it.

Your restored body, renewed mind, and revived spirit were never just for you. They were always meant to overflow—to your family, your circle, your community, and into your calling.

So, let the last word of this journey not be an ending... but an invitation:

> To become the sanctuary others need,
>
> To speak truth where silence has lingered,
>
> To walk with others the same way the Creator has walked with you.

Because Eden was never meant to stay lost.

It was meant to be lived, shared, and multiplied.

And the garden... is just beginning to grow again.

II. The Wounds of Disconnection

Trauma often happens in relationships, but so does restoration.

Loneliness as an Inflammatory, Emotional Burden

When trust is broken, self-protection builds walls instead of bridges.

If Eden was designed for connection, then the great wound of the fall was disconnection—from YHVH, from each other, from the land, and even from ourselves.

Where the Wound Begins

Trauma doesn't occur in a vacuum. It most often originates in a relationship through betrayal, neglect, abuse, abandonment, or emotional absence. We were made for safety in connection, so when that safety is violated, the pain runs deep.

And because wounds often occur through relationships, true healing also requires a relationship—the kind that is slow, safe, and rooted in grace.

But many of us have tried to survive that pain by building invisible walls:

> Walls of independence: "I don't need anyone."

> Walls of silence: "I'm fine."

> Walls of performance: "If I'm perfect, I won't be rejected."

These walls protect us from further hurt… but they also keep out healing.

Loneliness Is More Than Sadness —It's Inflammation

We often underestimate the cost of isolation. It's not just emotional—it's physical. Scientific research now confirms what Scripture hinted at all along: "…It is not good for man to be alone..." (Genesis 2:18).

Loneliness is now recognized as a serious public health issue. According to a 2023 advisory from the U.S. Surgeon General, loneliness increases the risk of:

> Heart disease by 29%,

> Stroke by 32%,

Dementia by 50%,

Premature death at a rate comparable to smoking 15 cigarettes a day (U.S. Department of Health and Human Services, 2023).

In a study published in Proceedings of the National Academy of Sciences, researchers found that loneliness triggers increased activity in genes associated with inflammation and suppressed immune function (Cole, 2015).

Loneliness isn't just an ache in the soul—it's a burden on the body.

The Cost of Broken Trust

When trust has been broken, especially in spiritual or intimate relationships, our nervous system often shifts into a state of permanent defense. Even small moments of vulnerability can feel dangerous.

We may:

Avoid the community altogether,

Mask emotions to appear strong,

Assume rejection before it happens,

Distrust even those who seem safe and try to help.

But Eden cannot be rebuilt on the soil of suspicion. It requires courage to reenter connection: first with YHVH, then with ourselves, and finally with others.

From Walls to Bridges

The invitation of this chapter is not to deny the hurt. It's to move from walls to bridges slowly.

That begins with:

> Naming the wound,
>
> Inviting YHVH into the place of pain,
>
> Letting someone who feels safe to see the real you,
>
> Practicing relational rhythms (like shared meals, prayer, conversation),
>
> Asking for help when you'd rather hide.

Because when we begin to feel safe again, our body relaxes. Our immune system rebalances. Our nervous system exhales. And healing—true, Edenic healing—begins to multiply.

You Were Never Meant to Heal Alone

> Disconnection is the wound.
>
> Connection is the cure.
>
> And the garden is waiting to be rebuilt—together.

III. Building an Edenic Circle

Spiritual Friendships vs. Codependent Entanglements

Healing is deeply personal, but it's not meant to stay private.

YHVH didn't just form Adam. He created Eve. He blessed their union, charged them with purpose, and built a garden not only of life, but of relationship. The Edenic blueprint always included shared presence, mutual support, and sacred togetherness.

If we want to sustain the healing we've cultivated in solitude, we must bring it into community. But not just any community—a circle that reflects Eden's peace and YHVH's presence.

What a Safe Community Looks Like

A healthy, Edenic circle is not based on perfection. It is rooted in honesty, grace, truth, and mutual growth. It's a space where:

Vulnerability is met with compassion

Correction is given in love, not control

Emotions are acknowledged, not dismissed

Success is celebrated, not compared

Struggles are shared, not shamed

Everyone contributes something, and no one carries everything

This kind of circle becomes a greenhouse for growth. It's where spiritual practices can be embodied and emotional safety nurtured.

Spiritual Friendship vs. Codependent Entanglement

Not all "Christian" or "faith-based" communities are Edenic. Some groups operate out of fear, driven by performance or power imbalances. That's not restoration—it's religious captivity.

Let's clarify the difference:

Spiritual Friendship	Codependent Entanglement
Freely given support	Conditional involvement
Encourages independence in YHVH	Requires emotional caretaking
Holds space without judgment	Fixes, rescues, or controls
Speaks truth in love	Avoids truth to keep peace
Grows both people	Drains or disempowers one party

Edenic relationships are anchored in freedom. They point each other to YHVH, not to self. They provide safety without becoming a substitute for the Spirit.

Sharing Meals, Worship, and Rest in Rhythm

One of the simplest (and most powerful) ways to build community is by breaking bread together.

Invite others for a plant-based Sabbath meal

Start a weekly worship circle in your home or online

Create a safe space for others to pray, cry, and heal

Observe rest days or tech-free hours together

Practice gratitude, scripture reading, or outdoor walks in community

These rhythms aren't just habits—they are acts of resistance against the isolation of modern life. They say: We were not made to rush. We were not made to hide. We were made to walk together in truth and peace.

Rebuilding Eden Together

No one can do this alone, and you're not meant to.

If you've healed quietly, that's beautiful. But now is the time to gather, to open your table, and to be part of someone else's restoration.

Even just one safe person can become the start of an Edenic circle. A garden doesn't grow overnight, but it grows together.

IV. Accountability and Intercession

Confess, pray, and stand in the gap for one another—because spiritual warfare, declarations, and healing were never meant to be done alone; they require the courage to be both vulnerable and powerful simultaneously.

Healing may begin in solitude, but it grows roots in shared soil.

When we choose to walk in Edenic community, we reclaim more than support—we reclaim intercession, accountability, and shared authority. These are not spiritual accessories. They are the scaffolding of lasting transformation.

Confess, Pray, and Stand Together

Scripture speaks clearly: "Confess therefore your sins one to another, and pray one for another, that ye may be healed. The supplication of a righteous man availeth much in its working," (James 5:16).

There is healing in confession—not just vertically to YHVH, but horizontally in a trusted community. This doesn't mean sharing your story with anyone and everyone. It means discerning safe people who will:

> Listen without judgment,

> Pray with intention and discernment,

> Point you back to truth,

> Stand in the gap when you feel too weak to fight.

When you know someone is praying for you by name—covering your health, your emotions, your mind, your family—it changes everything. It lightens the spiritual load. It reminds you that you are not alone.

Spiritual Warfare Isn't Meant to Be Solo

Warfare is real, but it was never designed to be done in isolation. In Eden, there was no warfare. However, after the fall, we now face battles in thought, emotion, and atmosphere. Thankfully, we do not fight alone.

Together, we can:

> Declare the truth when someone is battling lies,

> Fast for a breakthrough in another's health or household,

Rebuke fear, shame, and confusion in unity,

Use anointed prayers and scripture to reclaim peace,

Sing, speak, and shout declarations of life over each other.

This kind of shared warfare shifts atmospheres. It breaks spiritual inertia. And it reminds the enemy that we are not easy prey! We are restored image-bearers, standing shoulder to shoulder in sacred authority!

Vulnerable and Powerful — At the Same Time

The world teaches that strength is often found in silence. That vulnerability equals weakness. But in the Kingdom? It's the opposite.

You can be vulnerable and powerful at the same time.

You can say, "I'm struggling," and still cast out fear.

You can cry during prayer and still speak healing over someone else.

You can feel broken and still be used to bring restoration.

That's what Edenic community looks like.

It's not about being perfect. It's about being present, transparent, and committed to each other's healing.

The Commission of Community

You were never meant to just "get better" and move on.

You were meant to get free and help others do the same.

Be the one who checks in.

Be the one who gently asks the deeper question.

Be the one who says, "I'm not letting you quit."

Be the one who prays with fire and hugs with tenderness.

This is how Eden spreads—not just through ideas, but through interwoven lives, grounded in truth and alive in the Spirit.

Because restoration, when shared, becomes revival.

V. Creating Spaces of Healing for Others

Your healing becomes a seed for someone else's.

Leading a small group, hosting a meal, or simply listening can restore Eden for someone else.

Being Willing to Be Seen, Known, and Sent

Eden isn't just a place you return to for yourself.

It's a place you recreate—for others.

Every step of your healing—each lie renounced, each habit broken, each tear shed and exchanged for peace—becomes a living testimony. A seed. A sacred ripple in the lives of those around you.

When you walk in restoration, you don't just shine…

You light the path for someone still stuck in darkness.

Your Healing Is Someone Else's Breakthrough

You don't need a title, a stage, or a degree.

You need a table, a little time, and a heart that says "yes."

Healing flows most powerfully through simple acts of hospitality:

Hosting a meal that nourishes bodies and opens hearts,

Starting a small group where people can be honest and rooted in truth,

Creating a safe space for someone to cry, confess, and exhale,

Sharing your story—not when it's perfect, but when it's honest.

When someone sees that you were once where they are—and that transformation is possible—they begin to hope again. They start to believe that Eden isn't just for other people. It's for them, too.

Restoration as Reproduction

The fruit of Eden was never meant to be hoarded. It was meant to multiply.

When you live Eden out loud—through your habits, your hospitality, your healed mindset—you model a new way of being:

A home with peace instead of chaos,

A body treated with respect instead of neglect,

A soul anchored in truth instead of tossed by trauma,

A spirit that knows when to rest, when to war, and when to worship.

This isn't about perfection. It's about presence. When you offer presence to others—without judgment, without rushing, without fixing—you create space for the Ruach to move.

Be Seen, Be Known, Be Sent

There is risk in stepping out. Risk in being seen. Risk in saying, "This is who I am now. This is what I've walked through." But that's how the Kingdom grows.

Eden is restored every time someone:

> Says "yes" to being vulnerable,
>
> Says "yes" to creating a safe space,
>
> Says "yes" to being sent into homes, hospitals, coffee shops, and congregations with nothing but compassion, conviction, and connection.

You don't need a perfect house to host healing.

You don't need perfect words to speak life.

You just need the courage to show up—whole-hearted, Spirit-filled, and Eden-minded.

This Is How the Garden Grows

Eden doesn't grow because you've mastered it.

It grows because you're willing to share it.

Your life becomes the soil.

Your testimony becomes the seed.

And YHVH brings the increase.

So, go.

Be seen.

Be known.

Be sent.

And let healing multiply through you.

13—Creation Heals: Returning to the Natural World

When YHVH planted a garden in Eden, He didn't place humanity in a temple, a classroom, or a gym. He placed us in a living ecosystem. Eden was alive with color, movement, sound, scent, and light. The trees weren't just for food. The rivers weren't only for watering the land. Every element of Eden spoke to the body, mind, and spirit. Creation itself was part of the design for health and connection.

We were made to dwell in the natural world. And when we distance ourselves from it, something in us forgets how to breathe.

I. The Physiology of Reconnection

Modern science is finally catching up with ancient wisdom: nature heals.

Forest Bathing and Nervous System Calm

The Japanese practice of shinrin-yoku, or "forest bathing," is the simple act of spending time among trees. Research shows it reduces cortisol (the stress hormone), lowers heart rate and blood pressure, and activates the parasympathetic nervous system—the part of us that is responsible for rest and digestion (Park, 2010).

Grounding and Cellular Balance

When we walk barefoot on natural ground—soil, sand, rocks, grass— our bodies absorb free electrons from the earth. These electrons have been shown to reduce inflammation, improve sleep, and balance circadian rhythms (Chevalier, 2012). Grounding isn't just relaxing; it's regulating at a cellular level.

Circadian Rhythms and Sunlight

Sunlight signals the brain to regulate the production of melatonin and serotonin. A lack of natural light is directly linked to sleep disorders, depression, and hormonal imbalances (Cajochen, 2007). Eden had no fluorescent bulbs. Just the rhythm of the sun and moon, in perfect sync with the body's own rhythms.

The Power of Fresh Air

Air filled with negative ions—found near waterfalls, mountains, and forests—improves oxygen absorption, stabilizes mood, and increases alertness (Pierce, 2011). No wonder the garden was the perfect home for Adam and Eve. Even the air was medicine.

II. Gardening: Therapy and Spiritual Discipline

Gardening is not just a hobby—it's a holy act. When you put your hands in the soil, you remember your origin, as Genesis 3:19 informs: from the dust you were taken. Working the ground connects you with creation, the Creator, and self.

Gardening as grounding: Tending the soil has been shown to decrease anxiety and depression. Certain soil bacteria (Mycobacterium vaccae) even act as natural antidepressants (Lowry, 2007).

Spiritual parallel: Just as we prune plants, YHVH prunes our hearts. Just as seeds need water and light, we need Word and Spirit. The lessons of the soil are divine metaphors waiting to be lived.

Provision and purpose: In Eden, Adam was not idle. He was a steward of the garden (Genesis 2:15). Gardening restores that call.

III. Nature Reflects the Voice of the Creator

"The heavens declare the glory of God;
And the firmament showeth his handiwork.
[2] Day unto day uttereth speech,
And night unto night showeth knowledge," (Psalm 19:1-2).

The natural world doesn't whisper—it shouts the truth of YHVH's goodness. When we immerse ourselves in His creation, we remember what's real:

> The cycle of seasons mirrors the cycles of healing and rest.
>
> The beauty of wildflowers reminds us that we are clothed without striving.
>
> The birds that sing at dawn tell us worry is wasted energy (Matthew 6:26).
>
> The sound of rushing water echoes His voice that thunders with life (Revelation 1:15).

We don't just encounter nature—we hear the Creator's voice through it. The garden is still speaking.

IV. Returning to Eden Through Creation

You don't need to move to a cabin in the woods to return to Eden. But you do need to reintroduce creation into your rhythm.

Simple Ways to Reconnect:

> Sit outside barefoot for 15 minutes a day—no phone.
>
> Grow something edible in a pot or garden—tomatoes, herbs, greens.
>
> Watch the sunrise once a week. Let the light recalibrate your body.
>
> Replace synthetic smells with real ones: lemon zest, rosemary, fresh dirt.
>
> Go for a walk near trees. Breathe in slowly and listen.

This is not self-care. It's soul care. It's Eden care.

V. The Garden Was Always Part of the Plan

In Revelation 22, the story comes full circle: the Tree of Life stands again, bearing fruit each month, and the leaves are for the healing of the nations. The garden wasn't a temporary paradise. It was a pattern—a template for healing, nourishment, and connection.

Creation still heals. Eden still lives. And you were made to walk with your Creator among the trees.

VI. Creation and Emotional Regulation

While the body responds physiologically to the natural world, the soul responds emotionally. Modern life overstimulates the nervous system with screens, synthetic light, and noise pollution, but creation offers the opposite: calm, clarity, and comfort.

Beauty as Emotional Medicine

Studies show that viewing natural beauty—like flowers, sunsets, and water—stimulates the production of dopamine, the brain's "feel good" chemical (Zhang, 2014) (Zeki, 2014). This isn't accidental. Beauty is a signature of the Creator. It doesn't just please the eye; it heals the heart.

Stillness for Inner Stability

Being in nature quiets the internal dialogue. The rustling of leaves, the chirping of birds, and the distant hum of bees offer a soundscape that reduces internal noise. Psalm 46:10 says, "Be still and know that I am God." Stillness isn't passive—it's powerful. It realigns you with Presence.

Nature as Safe Attachment

Trauma-informed studies suggest that those who've experienced emotional neglect or attachment wounds often find security and comfort in animals, trees, and open skies. These elements don't judge, criticize, or abandon—they hold you. Nature becomes what therapist and author Linda Buzzell calls a "trustworthy presence," offering a sense of safety where human relationships may have failed (Buzzell, 2009).

This phenomenon is echoed in ecotherapy research, where natural environments are shown to serve as a "holding space" for emotional healing, especially in children and adults affected by trauma (Berger, 2010) (Jordan, 2016).

Similarly, animals have been found to foster attachment-like bonds and regulate stress in those with emotional wounds, providing companionship that bypasses the complexity of human relationships (Fine, 2015). In many ways, creation re-parents the parts of us that never learned peace, offering the nervous system a calm, secure base for restoration (Porges, 2011).

VII. Digital Overload vs. Divine Design

We live in a world that is visually overstimulating and spiritually under-nourishing. Digital screens demand attention but offer little in the way of restoration. Creation, on the other hand, invites reflection and offers renewal.

The Opposite of Eden

Scrolling isn't the same as seeing. Digital environments are often designed for addiction, not alignment. While Eden spoke in rhythms and seasons, screens speak in alerts and interruptions. To return to creation is to reclaim agency over your attention.

Micro-Sabbaths in Nature

Not everyone can take long retreats, but everyone can build small, daily respites. Even five minutes watching the wind in the trees is a holy pause. These micro-Sabbaths help recalibrate your soul and shift your energy from scattered to settled.

Neuroplasticity Through Nature

Just as negative digital habits can wire the brain for stress and distraction, intentional time in nature can rewire it for peace, gratitude, and a sense of awe. A single intentional walk outdoors has been shown to reduce rumination—the cycle of negative thoughts—and increase creative problem-solving (Bratman, 2015).

VIII. Children and Creation: Restoring Wonder Early

Our children are growing up indoors—under artificial lights, behind screens, disconnected from dirt, trees, and animals. This isn't just unfortunate; it's devastating! It's forming their brains and souls in a way that deviates from the divine design.

Developmental Need, Not Luxury

Nature play enhances motor skills, strengthens the immune system, boosts confidence, and reduces ADHD symptoms (Kuo, 2004). But even more, it nurtures a sense of wonder, and wonder is the foundation of worship.

Teach Through Tending

Inviting children to garden, care for animals, or observe the weather isn't only educational—it's formative. They learn patience through seasons, responsibility through watering, and joy through the miracle of life. These are the original "object lessons" of the Garden.

IX. Creation and Worship: Rekindling Awe

Creation was never meant to be worshipped, but it was always meant to lead us to worship.

"…Stand still, and consider the wondrous works of God," (Job 37:14).

Each leaf, wave, and breeze is a testimony. They don't speak Hebrew or Greek, but they declare His glory in a universal tongue. When you pause long enough to really *see* creation, you begin to feel what Adam must have felt: a heart wide open, reverent, and aware.

Simple Practices to Rekindle Awe:

Wake early to bless the rising sun with gratitude.

Light a candle and pray outside as evening falls.

Journal beside a tree or running water.

Memorize Psalm 104 and speak it aloud under the sky.

Bless the food you grow, and the soil that nurtured it.

These aren't rituals for ritual's sake. They are realignments—soul posture adjustments—that remind us: *we are creatures, not creators,* and the Garden is still whispering its invitation.

X. Rewilding the Soul

The deeper truth is this: Eden never left us. We left Eden. But the memory of it is written in our cells, in our lungs, in our longing for more than concrete and chaos.

> To walk barefoot again.
> To drink clean water again.
> To sit in silence and feel *held* again.

This is not a hobby. It's healing. Not just for the body, but for the soul.

Rewilding isn't rebellion—it's return. A return to your origin. A return to the rhythm of rest, reverence, and relationship.

"They heard the voice of YHVH Elohim walking in the garden in the cool of the day..." (Genesis 3:8).
That voice still walks.
That garden still heals.
And your soul still remembers the way.

14—Planting Eden in the Next Generation

❦ ❦

"⁶ And these words, which I command thee this day, shall be upon thy heart; ⁷ and thou shalt teach them diligently unto thy children, and shalt talk of them when thou sittest in thy house, and when thou walkest by the way, and when thou liest down, and when thou risest up," (Deuteronomy 6:6-7).

Eden wasn't meant to stop with us.

The restoration we pursue in our bodies, emotions, and spirits is not just a personal journey—it's a generational legacy. If Eden is being restored in our homes, then our children should be the first ones to taste its fruit.

This chapter is not about perfect parenting. It's about planting seeds. Seeds of truth.

Seeds of peace.

Seeds of life.

Seeds that, when nurtured with presence and grace, grow into generations that walk with YHVH in the cool of the day.

I. A Home That Feels Like Eden

Children thrive in environments that echo the rhythms of Eden:

Safety

Simplicity

Nourishment

Rest

Connection

Create a Home of:

Nourishment – Teach them that food is not just fuel, but worship. Involve them in planting, chopping, tasting, and blessing. Let meals be slow and sacred.

Rest – Prioritize peace. Set boundaries that protect quiet, rest, and sleep. Model unplugging. Sabbath is one of the greatest gifts you can pass on.

Truth – Speak truth over your children often. Help them identify lies early:

"You're not enough."

"You have to earn love."

"You're bad when you feel angry."

Replace lies with YHVH's declarations.

Presence – More than toys, children need your eye contact, your listening, your laughter. Being present is how they learn they're worth loving.

Order and Wonder – Let them participate in the beauty of a tidy, rhythm-filled home. A peaceful space speaks safety to the nervous system. Let art supplies, nature treasures, and Scripture reminders be more accessible than screens or noise.

They don't need a perfect home. They need a rooted one.

II. Protecting Developing Minds

Children today face a flood of toxins—many invisible, yet deeply formative.

What to Guard Them From:

> **Food toxins** – Artificial dyes, preservatives, processed sugar, and seed oils don't just harm bodies. They impact behavior, focus, and emotional regulation. Multiple studies show links between food additives and ADHD, mood dysregulation, and even aggression (Stevens, 2013).

> **Media toxins** – Screens filled with violence, sexual content, anxiety-fueling messages, and rapid dopamine spikes wire children's brains for overstimulation and despair. They shape what your child desires.

> **Spiritual toxins** – Just like unclean food, unclean spiritual

environments leave residue. Teach discernment early. Help them know the voice of the Good Shepherd from a counterfeit.

Environmental toxins – The body absorbs what's in the air, water, and home. Prioritize non-toxic cleaning products, filtered water, and natural fibers. Your choices shape their baseline of normal.

Be proactive, not paranoid. Explain why your family lives differently—not out of fear, but out of faith. Equip them to choose Eden when Babylon offers them candy.

*See The Eden Way Toolbox for a checklist.

III. Teaching Rhythms of Eden Early

Children don't learn from lectures. They learn from life. That means the best way to pass on Edenic values is by living them—out loud and in rhythm.

Teach Through:

Sabbath – Let them help light candles, sing songs, and prep food. Make Sabbath fun. Not legalistic, but life-giving.

Gardening – Even one pot of basil or a tray of microgreens lets kids witness the miracle of creation and stewardship.

Scripture – Don't just read verses. Live them. Tie them to daily moments: kindness on the playground, prayers at bedtime, and awe at the stars.

Gratitude – Make thankfulness a game. Share "top 3 blessings" each night. Sing your thanks. Draw them. Laugh about them. Gratitude plants roots.

Movement and Rest – Dance with your kids. Lie under the sky. Let them see that rest is as holy as productivity—and both belong to YHVH.

Consecrated Words – Teach them the sacredness of the Name YHVH. Help them speak blessings, not curses. Let their language be shaped by light, not sarcasm or shame.

IV. Healing the Parent to Raise the Child

Let's be honest: many of us are still re-parenting ourselves. We carry patterns from our own upbringing—some helpful, some hurtful. To raise Edenic children, we must first let YHVH restore us.

Heal Through:

Grace – Forgive your younger self. Forgive your parents. Forgive your moments of snapping, yelling, withdrawing. Eden isn't about perfection. It's about return.

Awareness – Ask yourself: What did I need as a child? What do I wish someone had taught me? Then give that gift—first to yourself, then to your children.

Intention – Be deliberate in creating rhythms. It's never too late. Even grown children can witness your transformation and be changed by it.

Repair – Don't be afraid to apologize. Restoration is not about never failing. It's about returning with humility and trying again. Modeling healthy repair teaches them trust and grace.

Your wholeness makes room for theirs. Every healed response you model, every fear you bring to YHVH, every choice to stay present plants a seed of Eden in their spirit.

The Garden Is Meant to Grow

You are not just restoring Eden—you are replanting it.

In every story you tell, every prayer you speak, every meal you make, and every tear you wipe… you're sowing seeds that will outlive you.

So, take heart. The garden may begin with you, but it doesn't have to end there.

"Lo, children are a heritage of Jehovah; *And* the fruit of the womb is *his* reward," (Psalm 127:3).

Let's raise them to remember the garden. And one day, to restore it even further than we did.

Sabbath Activity Guide for Kids

Helping Children Experience the Joy of Shabbat
Designed for ages 4–12 but adaptable for younger or older children, this guide helps children engage with the beauty, peace, and joy of Shabbat while honoring its purpose as a set-apart time of rest and connection.

Friday Night Prep (Erev Shabbat)

Let kids take part in setting the tone and space for rest.

Activities:

- o *Shabbat Table Helper:* Set the table with candles, flowers, or handmade placemats.
- o *Candle Lighting:* Teach the meaning behind the candles. Let them hold a flameless one.
- o *Blessing Cards:* Create or color blessings for parents, siblings, or guests.
- o *"Shabbat Snack Plate":* Arrange grapes, nuts, olives, figs, or a special treat.

Shabbat Morning

Begin with a slow, joy-filled rhythm.

Activities:

- o *Morning Song & Stretch:* Sing "Shabbat Shalom" or a calming worship song.
- o *"Thank You" Nature Walk:* Name five things to thank YHVH for in creation.
- o *Sabbath Storytime:* Read from the Bible—Creation, Manna, or Yeshua healing.
- o *Create a "Rest Nest":* Cozy reading and worship corner with pillows and blankets.

Creative Quiet Time

Offer calm expression options.

Activities:

- *Coloring Pages:* Candles, stars, trees, animals, or Psalm 23 themes.
- *Draw "What Peace Feels Like":* Encourage imagination and expression.
- *Sabbath Journal:* Write or draw thank-you's to YHVH.
- *Build Eden with LEGOs:* Create trees, rivers, and gardens.

Afternoon Peace Activities

Encourage gentle play and connection.

Ideas:

- *"Peaceful People" Charades:* Act out a shepherd, baker, gardener, or dove.
- *Gratitude Chain:* Add a thankful paper link each week.
- *Bubble Prayers:* Blow bubbles while whispering prayers of thanks.
- *Shabbat Blessing Circle:* Bless each other with a few heartfelt words.

Suggested Sabbath Read-Aloud Books

- *Psalm 23* (child-friendly versions)
- *The Very Quiet Cricket* by Eric Carle
- *All-of-a-Kind Family* by Sydney Taylor (classic Sabbath scenes)
- *A Child's Book of Blessings* by Sabrina Dearborn
- *The Peace Rose* by Alicia Jewell or any gentle story emphasizing kindness and rest.
- *Shabbat is here!* (Poem located in the back of the book in The Eden Way Toolbox)

o   *The Keeper and the Seeds of Truth* by Angel Tate Keaton (Coming Soon)

Optional Preparation Tools for Parents

o   "Sabbath Box" with quiet crafts, toys, and Scripture
o   Pre-printed blessings or memory verses
o   Calm worship playlist or nature sounds
o   Kid-friendly prayer and declaration cards
o   A special Shabbat table runner made by your kids

As we plant seeds of Eden in the hearts of our children, we're not just raising boys and girls—we're raising image-bearers, future restorers, and carriers of covenant. Every small choice to model love, truth, peace, and wonder is a holy act of generational healing. The garden may begin in our homes, but its branches will stretch far beyond us—into classrooms, neighborhoods, communities, and the world. So, we water what we've planted with grace, we guard it with prayer, and we trust the Gardener to bring the increase. Eden lives on… because we chose to continue planting those seeds.

15—Grieving What Was Lost: When Healing Includes Lament

🌿🌿

"Blessed are they that mourn: for they shall be comforted," (Matthew 5:4).

Eden was a place of beauty, connection, and abundance, but it was also a place that was lost. And before we can fully restore what was, we must grieve for what no longer is.

Many people attempt healing through food, mindset, or spiritual disciplines while unknowingly dragging behind them a heavy cloak of unprocessed grief.

If we do not stop to mourn, we carry our wounds into every attempt at restoration. Healing cannot be forced on top of buried pain. Like seeds, healing grows best in soil softened by tears.

I. Grieving the Body You Abused or Neglected

Before restoration can take root in your physical body, you must acknowledge what your body has been through, especially when you were the one who harmed it, even unintentionally.

You May Be Mourning:

> Years of disordered eating, crash diets, or emotional eating.
>
> Seasons of overwork or burnout, ignoring your body's need for rest.
>
> Medical decisions you made in desperation or by trusting a system that failed you.
>
> The simple loss of innocence about how beautiful and good your body was created to be.

Let yourself lament. Talk to your body like a friend you once neglected. Say you're sorry. And then promise to do better from a place of grace, not guilt.

II. Grieving Betrayal, Church Wounds, and Childhood Trauma

So much of our pain is not physical—it's relational. Betrayal by those we once trusted, wounds from spiritual leaders, and the scars left by our earliest experiences create strongholds that block healing.

> What This Grief Can Look Like:
>
> Anger that turns inward as shame.
>
> Silence and avoidance to avoid reopening wounds.

Perfectionism that tries to "outperform" the pain.

But grief doesn't go away when ignored. It leaks. It festers. It transforms into depression, anxiety, or even autoimmune conditions. That's why Scripture doesn't just show us healing. It also shows us lament.

> "Thou numberest my wanderings:
> Put thou my tears into thy bottle;
> Are they not in thy book" (Psalm 56:8)?

III. The Role of Tears in Detox and Healing

Tears are not weakness—they are a sacred release.

Tears are more than an emotional expression—they play a biochemical role in stress relief. Research by biochemist William Frey found that emotional tears (as opposed to reflex tears) contain stress-related substances like adrenocorticotropic hormone (ACTH) and manganese, suggesting that crying may help the body eliminate toxins and reduce stress through a form of biochemical detoxification (Frey, 1985).

Furthermore, crying has been shown to activate the parasympathetic nervous system, leading to lowered heart rate and a calming effect on the body (Vingerhoets, 2016). This means that crying is not only a psychological release, but it also supports physiological recovery.

Grief softens the heart and clears space in the nervous system for rest and repair.

So, cry. Not just once, but whenever the ache surfaces. Let lament be part of your Eden journey.

IV. Scriptural Laments: Models for Emotional Release

YHVH doesn't shame grief. He models how to do it well.

Examples of Scriptural Lament:

> David cried out in the Psalms, asking "Why have You forsaken me?" yet ending with hope. (Psalm 22:24–31)

> Jeremiah poured out deep sorrow in Lamentations over a broken Jerusalem. (Lamentations 1:16; 2:11; 3:48–50)

> Even Yeshua wept—over Lazarus, over Jerusalem, and in Gethsemane. (John 11:35; Luke 19:41; Matthew 26:38–39; Luke 22:44, respectively)

Lament is not a lack of faith. It is honest worship in its rawest form.

Use the Psalms as a guide. Pray them aloud. Rewrite them in your journal in your own words. Let them give your grief structure and sacred space.

V. A Safe Place to Weep

Grief must have a container—a safe space where tears are not rushed or explained away.

That may be:

> A journal and a candlelit corner

> A trusted friend who listens without fixing

> A Sabbath Walk where you talk aloud to YHVH

> A song that lets you sob until you're empty

Give yourself permission to mourn what could have been, what was lost, and what has not yet healed.

VI.   The Garden Included Sorrow

Eden was never meant to hold death or tears, but after the fall, sorrow became part of the human story.

And even in Revelation, when Eden is fully restored, one of the final promises is this:

"…and he shall wipe away every tear from their eyes; and death shall be no more; neither shall there be mourning, nor crying, nor pain, any more: the first things are passed away," (Revelation 21:4).

Tears are part of the return. They wash the soil of your soul and water the seeds of restoration.

So, cry. Grieve. Lament. And know this: even in your sorrow, you are walking the Eden path.

Lament Journal Prompt: Writing Your Own Psalm of Grief and Hope

"Out of the depths have I cried unto thee, O Jehovah," (Psalm 130:1).

The Psalms teach us that it's okay to bring our overflowing hearts to YHVH—including sorrow, confusion, fear, and pain. Writing your own psalm is not about sounding poetic—it's about being honest. It's about making space for grief and anchoring it to hope.

How to Write a Psalm of Lament

Most biblical psalms of lament follow this pattern:

1. Address YHVH

Call on Him by Name. Be personal. ("O YHVH…" or "Heavenly Father…")

2. State the Complaint or Grief

Be raw. Be honest. Tell YHVH what hurts, what confuses you, or what feels unfair.

3. Ask for Help

Request healing, justice, understanding, or peace. Be specific.

4. Express Trust or Hope

Shift into remembrance or expectation—even if it's small. Trust doesn't erase pain—it holds it.

5. Declare Praise

End with a sentence of faith, praise, or a declaration of His goodness—even if it's through tears.

Writing Prompts

Use these prompts to reflect, then turn your thoughts into your own Psalm below.

1. What am I grieving today?

What loss, pain, or wound still weighs on me?

2. What do I want to say to YHVH that I haven't said yet?

This can be anger, tears, confusion, or fear. Nothing is off limits.

3. What do I need from Him right now?

Comfort? Answers? Strength? A sign that He sees you?

4. What truth do I still believe about who He is?

Even just one thing you're holding onto.

5. How will I choose to trust again, even in the ache?

A declaration, a promise, or a whisper of hope.

*You'll find a guided Psalm-writing form in the Eden Way Toolbox at the back of this book—your invitation to pour out your heart like David did.

16—The Eden to Come: Longing for the Final Garden

🚶 🚶

"...in the midst of the street thereof. And on this side of the river and on that was the tree of life, bearing twelve *manner of* fruits, yielding its fruit every month: and the leaves of the tree were for the healing of the nations," (Revelation 22:2).

From the very beginning, Eden was the pattern. It was never merely a garden. It was a sanctuary of wholeness. No shame. No sickness. No disconnection. A place where heaven and earth touched. And though Eden was lost, Scripture assures us: Eden is not gone. It is coming again.

The final pages of the Bible are not the end of the story. They are the beginning of the forever restoration. The promise of Eden restored isn't a fantasy. It's the fulfillment of everything YHVH intended when He spoke creation into being.

I.   The Tree of Life Reappears

Genesis begins with a garden and a tree of life. Revelation ends with that very tree once again bearing fruit year-round and healing the nations.

This is not poetry. This is prophecy.

The final chapters of Revelation unveil a renewed heaven and earth. There is no temple, because the presence of YHVH fills all. There is no night, because His light never fades. And there in the center flows the river of life, and beside it, the tree of life—restored, accessible, overflowing with nourishment.

In the Eden we lost, humanity was barred from the Tree. But in Eden restored, the Tree bears fruit for all nations and its leaves bring healing to every wound.

The Bible is a full-circle story. It begins in Eden. It ends in Eden restored.

But we're not there yet.

II.   Why Our Small Steps Still Matter

It's easy to ask, "If Eden is coming, why bother now?"

Because every act of restoration we make now is prophetic: It testifies that we believe Eden is real and that we will one day return to it. It is a reminder that the brokenness around us is not the final word. It shouts that YHVH is a Creator who restores, not abandons.

These choices are not cosmetic. They are covenantal.

When you eat nourishing, plant-based food...

    You proclaim that life is sacred, not disposable.

When you set aside Sabbath rest...

You declare trust in a coming age where striving will cease.

When you speak words of blessing and truth…

You reflect the purity that will fill the New Jerusalem.

When you choose forgiveness over resentment…

You echo the mercy that will define the world to come.

These small choices are not about legalism or perfection—they are a prophetic witness to a Kingdom that is both coming and already among us.

III. The Tension of "Now and Not Yet"

We live between two gardens—the one behind us and the one before us.

This is what the prophets longed for. Isaiah spoke of a day when the wolf would lie down with the lamb (Isaiah 11:6). Ezekiel described water flowing from the Temple bringing life to everything it touched (Ezekiel 47). Joel promised that YHVH would restore the years the locust had eaten (Joel 2:25). Amos envisioned mountains dripping with sweet wine (Amos 9:13). These weren't just metaphors. They were glimpses of the Eden to come.

We live in the overlap:

healed but still healing,

redeemed but still broken,

awake but still weary.

This tension isn't failure. It's faith.

"For the earnest expectation of the creation waiteth for the revealing of the sons of God," (Romans 8:19).

Even creation groans for Eden to be restored. We feel that same ache in our bones, our emotions, and our prayers. And yet, even now, we see glimpses.

> Moments of peace.

> Plates of healing food.

> Tears turned into worship.

> A neighbor forgiven.

> A family reconciled.

> A body finally nourished after years of neglect.

These are echoes of what is to come.

IV. Living Prophetically: Eden Now

You are not just healing for your own sake. You are becoming a signpost. A seed planter. A whisper of what's coming.

Eden living is:

🌿 🌿 Choosing simplicity in a world of noise

🌿 🌿 Practicing rest in a world that worships hustle

🌿 🌿 Feeding the body with life, not death

🌿 🌿 Nurturing the spirit with truth, not fear

🌿 🌿 Creating peace in your home when the world is in chaos

This isn't about striving to recreate paradise—it's about embodying the values of Eden, so when the final Garden comes, your soul is already familiar.

You are rehearsing heaven.

You are preparing a people.

You are saying with your life, "Eden matters. And it's coming."

Even more, you are tasting Eden in advance. Every time you align with the Creator's design—every breath of stillness, every act of love, every truth you choose to believe—you step onto sacred ground.

V. The Table of the Kingdom

Yeshua said, "for I say unto you, I shall not drink from henceforth of the fruit of the vine, until the kingdom of God shall come," (Luke 22:18).

Yeshua is even waiting for the banquet.

And yet, he left us a taste—a table of remembrance. Not of his suffering, but of the Kingdom that will be.

The Eden to come is not only about restoration. It is about reunion. We will feast at a table where no one is missing. No more disease. No more shame. No more separation between heaven and earth.

Every time you nourish your body in alignment with that coming reality, you practice Kingdom living. Every time you refuse to bow to the culture of death, you declare your citizenship in the world to come.

VI. Why Not Now? Why Not Here?

If Eden will one day be fully restored…

If the Tree of Life will again heal the nations…

If sorrow and death will be swallowed up forever…

Then ask yourself this:

    Why not start now?

    Why not plant Eden in your home, your habits, your heart?

    Why not be a living preview of what is to come?

Let your choices point to the garden we've never forgotten.

Let your healing testify to the Healer.

Let your family witness your hope in action.

And let your life whisper to the world:

    Eden is not just behind us or before us.

    Eden begins here.

        In your kitchen.

        In your breath.

        In your relationships.

        In your rest.

And the day will come when we will see the Tree of Life again—together. Until then, keep walking like the Garden is just around the bend.

17—When Eden Feels Far: Staying Faithful in the Struggle

You started this journey with excitement. The vision of Edenic living lit a fire inside you. You made changes—perhaps radical ones. You felt clearer. Stronger. Closer to your purpose.

But now the path feels harder. The symptoms haven't entirely gone. Your family isn't on board. You're tired. And Eden? It feels far away again.

This chapter is for those moments.

I. Healing Isn't Linear

We want the road to be smooth. But the truth is: healing is a winding path. Progress often looks like spirals, not straight lines.

You might experience:

> Flare-ups of old symptoms,

> Emotional regression or mood swings,

> Moments of doubt, grief, or feeling stuck.

This doesn't mean you're failing. It means your body, mind, and spirit are peeling back deeper layers. Every detour is still part of the destination.

Think of healing like detox:

> Sometimes things get messier before they get better.

> Sometimes clarity follows chaos.

> Sometimes silence means your soul is rearranging itself.

Like the land lying fallow before a fruitful harvest, your pauses and regressions are part of a sacred cycle. YHVH is still working—even in the stillness, even in the dark.

Don't panic when it's not instant. Eden was not built in a day, and neither is your restoration.

Hold fast. What feels like a delay might actually be an invitation to dig deeper.

II. When Others Don't Come with You

Perhaps your spouse still eats processed food or animal flesh. Your friends mock your Sabbath. Your church community thinks your health changes are "extreme."

Few things test your endurance like walking a narrow path alone!

But Noah built an ark without public approval.

Moses walked into the wilderness before the crowd followed.

Yeshua retreated before revealing.

You're not behind. You're early!

Still, it hurts. The ache for community is real. And sometimes Eden means learning to be planted—even when no one else around you is willing or able to water you.

What to do:

Find even one ally—a friend, mentor, or group who supports your walk.

Join or create a community of like-minded believers who are also seeking Eden.

Pray for your family's hearts—and continue to model love without pressure.

Set boundaries with compassion: protect your healing without condemning theirs.

Remember: you're not responsible for their journey. You are only responsible for your own.

When others don't understand, don't shrink your Eden to fit their comfort. Instead, let your quiet consistency be a living testimony.

III. The Trap of Perfectionism

When healing becomes performance, it turns toxic.

You begin to feel shame for flare-ups. You scrutinize your every bite. You fear missing one supplement or skipping a journal day. THAT is not Eden. THAT is Egypt dressed in wellness clothes.

Perfectionism is not a fruit of YHVH's Spirit.

Healing was never supposed to be a checklist. It was meant to be communion—restoring a relationship with your body, your God, and your purpose.

Let yourself be human. Healing doesn't mean doing everything right all the time. Healing means staying rooted in grace. Your Creator is not grading your Edenic performance. He's walking with you in the cool of the day—even when you're limping.

> You are not behind schedule.

> You are not failing.

> You are learning what it means to be whole while still healing.

IV. How to Show Up When It's Hard

When motivation wanes, routines falter, and symptoms persist, how do you persevere?

Here's what faithfulness looks like on weary days:

Pray simply.

"Help me, Abba. I'm tired. Meet me here."

You don't need fancy words. You just need honesty.

Rest intentionally.

Take a Sabbath nap.

Unplug.

Breathe deeply.

Rest is resistance.

You don't have to earn rest—it's your birthright.

Keep one rhythm.

Maybe it's herbal tea.

A Psalm.

A 10-minute walk barefoot in the yard.

One thread is enough to stay tied to Eden. Don't let go of everything—hold onto something.

Speak life.

"I may feel broken, but I'm being rebuilt."

"I'm not done yet."

"…he who began a good work in you will perfect it…"

(Philippians 1:6).

Write it down.

> Journal your doubts,
>
> your prayers,
>
> your wins.

Sometimes your own words will preach back to you.

You don't have to conquer the mountain every day. Just take the next faithful step.

V. Rebuilding Trust: With YHVH and Your Body

Sometimes it's not the path that's hard—it's the relationship with the One who made it.

Perhaps you have prayed for healing and haven't yet seen it. Maybe you have followed all the steps and still feel broken. Possibly, you're angry at your body for "betraying" you. These are sacred tensions.

The invitation is not to force belief, but to let YHVH hold your questions.

Healing includes trust repairs:

> Trusting your body's wisdom again,
>
> Trusting that YHVH's timing is mercy, not punishment,
>
> Trusting that progress is happening even when you don't feel it.

Your body is not your enemy. It is your partner in restoration. And your Creator is not distant. He is forming you, molding you like a potter molds his vessel in this very wilderness.

You are not being punished. You are being prepared.

Every delay may be deepening something inside you: compassion, patience, courage, presence.

Don't waste the waiting. Let it strengthen the roots that your fruit will one day hang from.

Final Encouragement

Eden may feel far.

But remember: even when Adam and Eve were exiled from the garden, YHVH still clothed them. He walked with them. He remained close by.

He's near to you, too.

> Your body may tremble, but your spirit is being steadied.

> Your healing may feel slow, but roots grow in darkness.

> Your tears may fall silently, but they are counted like precious oil.

You are not alone in the garden-less places. He is still the Gardener.

Don't stop.

> Don't turn back.

> Don't measure your success by perfection.

Measure it by faithfulness.

Even if all you do today is breathe and whisper,

"I still believe Eden is possible,"

you are still on the path.

And that… is holy ground.

18—Stewarding Eden: Time, Money, and the Weight of Enough

🌿🌿

"And Jehovah God took the man, and put him into the garden of Eden to dress it and to keep it," (Genesis 2:15).

Healing is beautiful, but let's be honest—it can feel expensive. Not just financially, but emotionally and energetically. From organic produce to water filters to supplements and Sabbath meals, many people quietly wonder, "Can I afford to live this way?"

Others may feel equally bankrupt in time and energy. The pressure to do all the things: to cook from scratch, rest deeply, garden, journal, exercise, detox, and read Scripture…It can feel like too much.

But in Eden, there was no scarcity. No hoarding. No lack.

There was:

> Provision, without pressure.

> Abundance, without addiction.

> Rhythms, without rush.

Let's remember: Eden isn't about extravagance. It's about alignment.

You can live Edenic principles even with limited resources, energy, and a modest home.

The key is stewardship.

I. Budgeting for Wellness: Eden on a Modest Income

You don't need a $500 juicer or a $1,000 pantry overhaul to return to Eden. You need wisdom. Creativity. And willingness to shift your priorities from fast to faithful.

Edenic Budget Principles:

> Buy bulk over branded – Dry beans, grains, and produce stretch far and store well. They are also less expensive than canned.

> Cook simply – Eden was full of plants, not processed plant products. You don't need fancy recipes to nourish your body.

> Start small – Replace one toxic item per month (e.g., plastic, fragrance). Small changes compound.

> Invest in reusables – Cloth napkins, glass containers, and metal straws save over time and reduce waste.

> Grow what you can – Even herbs in a windowsill reconnect you to Eden's soil and soul.

One pot of lentils, one loaf of homemade bread, one fresh salad from your balcony garden—these are sacred acts of stewardship. You don't need a gourmet kitchen to host the presence of YHVH at your table.

"He that is faithful in a very little is faithful also in much: and he that is unrighteous in a very little is unrighteous also in much," (Luke 16:10).

Yeshua was saying here that if someone can be trusted with just a little, that person can also be trusted with abundance. Be faithful with the little first.

Need a Practical Tool to Put This into Action?

Turn to the Edenic Living Budgeting Worksheet in the Eden Way Toolbox at the back of this book. It's a simple, peaceful guide to help you align your spending with your values, reduce financial stress, and steward your resources with purpose.

II. Sabbath: Resetting Time and Breaking Work Addiction

In a culture that equates busyness with value, Sabbath feels radical. But it's the Edenic blueprint.

Sabbath is the Creator's weekly reminder that:

You are not a machine.

You are not what you produce.

You are already enough.

Sabbath is the Creator's gift that says:

You don't have to earn your worth.

Rest is productive.

There is always enough time when aligned with Him.

And when you stop producing, you're reminded you're still beloved.

Sabbath Breaks:

Time scarcity — reminds you you're not in charge of the clock.

Over functioning — helps you slow down and receive.

Workaholism — restores trust in YHVH's provision.

Sabbath isn't just a break. It's a reset of your priorities. It recalibrates your soul to Eden's rhythm.

The most potent healing comes when we stop doing and start being.

And in that sacred pause, we remember: enough was already built in.

III. Escaping Consumerism in the Wellness World

Even the wellness movement can become Babylon in disguise.

Endless ads tell you that healing requires the next product, the perfect diet, the newest superfood. But Eden was not a shopping cart—it was a garden.

Signs of Consumerism Creep:

Constant comparison to online influencers,

Shame about what you can't afford,

Obsession with buying instead of becoming.

The lie says: "You need more to be enough."

> The truth says: "You were made for Eden long before marketing existed."

You don't have to purchase Eden. You already have access to it.

Healing is in your breath.

> In your prayer.

> > In the dirt.

> > > In the Word.

> > > > And in the table.

Not on the next sale.

> Choose intentionality over accumulation.

> Choose contentment over consumption.

> Choose stewardship over striving.

IV. Making Peace with Small Beginnings

You might be eating lentils again this week.

You may still have plastic containers.

Your Sabbath may look like quiet time with a sandwich and Scripture, rather than a full feast.

But small doesn't mean insignificant.

Edenic truth:

> A mustard seed moves mountains. (Matthew 17:20; Luke 17:6)

A widow's oil sustained her household. (2 Kings 4:1-7)

A single loaf of bread fed thousands. (John 6:9–13; Matthew 14:13–21; Mark 6:30–44; Luke 9:10–17)

Don't despise small beginnings. They are often holier than we realize.

Every simple meal offered in love is a communion.

Every small act of obedience waters a seed.

You are planting Eden one step at a time.

You are building altars in your kitchen.

And YHVH sees.

He does not measure your offering by size, but by surrender.

V. Trading Scarcity for Trust

Scarcity says:

"I don't have enough."

"I'll never be able to afford what they can."

"I'm behind."

But trust says:

"My daily bread is enough."

"YHVH knows what I need before I ask."

"What I steward will multiply."

Affirmations for Edenic Provision:

"I release fear of not having enough."

"My Father is a Provider, not a punisher."

"I will not buy my worth. I will walk in it."

"I don't need everything. I need alignment."

Provision doesn't always show up in your bank account. Sometimes it's in a neighbor's gift, an unexpected sale, a secondhand blessing, or a new rhythm of simplicity that frees you from overwhelm.

YHVH's provision may not look like luxury,

but it will always be enough.

"The young lions do lack, and suffer hunger;

But they that seek Jehovah shall not want any good thing," (Psalm 34:10).

Practical Stewardship Reflections

What can I simplify this week to save money or time?

What rhythm (such as Sabbath preparation or batch cooking) could help me better steward my energy?

Where have I allowed comparison to steal my contentment?

How can I turn my current limitations into creativity?

What's one act of faith I can take this week, even if it's small?

Final Encouragement

Eden was not a palace. It was not glamorous. It was a garden.

Humble, abundant, and held in the hands of the Creator.

So is your life.

Whether your Eden looks like a rice-and-veggie bowl by candlelight or a thrifted Sabbath table, your obedience honors YHVH.

Stewarding time, money, and energy is not about perfection. It's about presence.

It's about trust that grows in small acts.

It's about contentment rooted in faith.

It's about tending your garden—however small—with joy and reverence.

Because in His presence, there is always enough.

19—Walking It Out: Testimonies, Tools, and Transformation

I. Real Stories of Edenic Renewal

Eden is not a theory. It's a path that can be walked again—not geographically, but in alignment.

This chapter is where the abstract becomes personal, and the spiritual becomes visible in lives restored, bodies renewed, minds rewired, and spirits reignited. The journey back to Eden is not a straight line. It's a daily return, a reordering of what was lost. And the most powerful evidence of its truth is the lives it transforms.

My Story: From Breakdown to Blueprint

I didn't write this book from a mountaintop. I wrote it from the midst of a war against inflammation, emotional pain, spiritual fatigue, and years of unknowingly living out of alignment with the Creator's design.

My body was screaming through eczema, nerve pain, brittle nails, hair loss, and constant exhaustion. Doctors prescribed creams and pills, but no one asked what I was eating, believing, or repeating in my thoughts.

It wasn't until I began removing dairy, processed foods, and toxic thinking that healing began. It was slow. Gentle. Like Eden, it came in rhythm, not in a rush. As I embraced a whole food plant-based diet, aligned my daily habits with Sabbath and rest, and stopped running from emotional pain, I began to heal. Not just my skin… but my soul.

This book is not a sermon. It's a survival guide turned healing manual. Because I know Eden is possible again—because I've lived it.

Testimony from My Husband, Todd

Before we started walking the Eden Way, I thought I was doing fine. I was always moving. I worked from sunup to sundown, pushing through the heat, the fatigue, the aches and pains. That's just what men do, right? Provide. Produce. Push forward.

But looking back now, I can see I wasn't thriving. I was worn out, running on fumes, carrying extra weight I didn't even realize was affecting everything—my energy, my mood, and even my intimacy and confidence as a man.

Since embracing the Eden lifestyle—plant-based eating, intentional rest, and spiritual alignment—I've experienced a transformation I didn't think was possible at my age.

The weight came off steadily, and I wasn't even dieting! I was just eating real food, the kind that fuels the body instead of dragging it down. My joints stopped hurting. My strength came back. I can work in the heat now without getting drained like before. I recover faster. I sleep deeper. I think clearer.

One of the biggest changes was honoring the Sabbath. At first, it was hard for me to slow down. I was used to going nonstop, always thinking there was something else I had to do. But now? I look forward to Shabbat. That one day a week has become a refuge. It's not just rest for my body—it's rest for my soul. I can breathe. I feel peace. My mind isn't racing. I've learned that stopping is not weakness—it's wisdom. Sabbath is also the fastest day of the week!

And our marriage? It's stronger. There's more connection. More laughter. More unity in how we live and lead our home.

I used to think health was about survival. Now I know it's about alignment: body, mind, and spirit working together the way the YHWH designed them. I'm not chasing youth. I'm walking in purpose, and I'm grateful every day that I get to do it alongside my wife, who believed in this path even when I wasn't sure.

Eden isn't just a place. It's a way of life. And I'm proof that it works.

— Todd Keaton

Others Who Reclaimed Wholeness

Christine's Journey —Mental Renewal After Trauma

After surviving a painful childhood and adult betrayal, Christine struggled with intrusive thoughts, panic attacks, and constant self-sabotage. She'd been in therapy for years but felt stuck in loops.

When she began tracking her thoughts, speaking truth-based declarations, and removing processed sugar and stimulants from her diet, things began to shift. Pairing Scripture meditation with whole food nourishment, she discovered that healing the brain was not separate from healing the gut. As inflammation decreased, so did anxiety.

Chrstine now teaches others how to break generational strongholds by starting with their food, their thoughts, and their spiritual authority.

Naomi's Sabbath Reset

Naomi was burnt out. A homeschooling mom of five, she had no time for herself and rarely felt spiritually connected. She confessed, "I was cooking and teaching Torah, but I was still angry, tired, and resentful."

The turning point came when she started honoring the Sabbath not just with meals, but with her entire schedule. She prepared early. Lit candles. Turned off notifications. Played worship music. And she rested…without guilt.

It transformed her home. Her children became calmer. Her digestion improved. Her mind quieted. Naomi discovered that Shabbat wasn't a ritual—it was medicine.

These stories echo a truth we all need to remember:

Eden was not destroyed. It was hidden,

waiting to be reclaimed by those willing to align.

Joyce's Story — A Cautionary Tale of Returning to Babylon

Joyce, my beloved mother-in-law (of blessed memory), suffered deeply from Sjögren's syndrome. The dry eyes, nerve pain, joint stiffness, and crushing fatigue were her constant companions. For two long years, she depended on a walker and had experienced multiple dangerous falls that forced her to sell her home and move in with us for her safety.

She had every reason to give up—but she didn't. At least not at first.

When we introduced her to the Edenic lifestyle—whole plant-based foods, daily prayer, rest, hydration, and natural remedies—she began to transform. Her walker stayed parked in the corner. She could walk again with steadiness. Her neuropathy lessened. Her pain decreased. She laughed more. She moved more freely. Even her eyes, once painfully dry, found some comfort.

Joyce was living proof that the body wants to heal when given the right conditions. For a while, she embraced it—drinking the green smoothies, enjoying nourishing soups, participating in Shabbat rest. We saw hope returning to her face.

But healing requires not only action, it requires continued surrender.

And eventually, something shifted.

The pull of old cravings—the meats, the processed foods, the sugary comfort snacks of Babylon—began whispering again. The memories of taste overpowered the memory of pain. And slowly, she stopped participating. She closed herself off in her room. She rejected the foods that were helping her heal. She said, "I just want to eat what I want again. I've eaten that way for 80 years; I'll keep eating that way until I die!" And she did.

Her physical decline was rapid and devastating. In a matter of weeks, her energy vanished. Her legs weakened. Her inflammation flared. The walker returned, then a wheelchair, and soon even bathroom visits required assistance. For the last three months of her life, she was completely bedbound and unable to eat solid foods. The healing path she had once walked—freely, joyfully—was abandoned. And so, her healing unraveled.

We loved her dearly. We still do. Sharing her story is not meant to shame, but to warn.

Because Babylon will always offer comfort food that kills.

It will tempt with nostalgia, with indulgence, with convenience.

But Eden calls us back—not to restriction, but to restoration.

Joyce's story reminds us: the Eden path works, but only when we stay on it.

Healing is not a one-time choice. It is a daily "yes" to life. To alignment. To obedience.

Her memory lives on in our journey. And her story is a sacred caution for anyone tempted to turn back.

"...I have set before thee life and death, the blessing and the curse: therefore, choose life, that thou mayest live, thou and thy seed..." Deuteronomy 30:19.

Let us not grow weary. Let us not trade our healing for a moment of comfort. Let us honor those who came before by choosing life today.

In loving memory of Joyce Keaton, whose journey reminds us that healing is sacred, and faithfulness to the path matters. May her story inspire others to choose life, one day at a time.

II. Practical Tools and Templates

Returning to Eden isn't just a concept—it's a lifestyle. Transformation happens when truth is applied, structure is embraced, and consistency creates space for renewal. This section provides the practical tools you need to walk out what you've read—to turn insight into habit, and revelation into rhythm.

These aren't meant to be rigid formulas but flexible frameworks. You don't need to do them perfectly. You simply need to be intentional.

1. Daily Rhythm Guides

Your days need Edenic structure. Not packed schedules, but purposeful flow. These guides help restore rhythm to body, mind, and spirit.

Morning: Set the Tone

Scripture meditation

Truth declaration

Light movement and hydration

Simple, whole food breakfast

Midday: Align and Refocus

Breath prayer or walk outside

Nourishing lunch

Journaling prompt (What am I feeling? Believing? Repeating?)

10-minute reset (music, rest, or stretch)

Evening: Release and Restore

Gratitude practice

Gentle dinner with family or quiet

No screens 1 hour before sleep

Prayer and reflection: What lie did I release today? What truth did I receive?

Sabbath Rhythm

Friday prep checklist

Special meals and table settings

Lighting candles and praying aloud

No to-do lists—yes to rest, connection, and delight

2. Edenic Recipes and Pantry Lists

Eating Edenically isn't about perfection—it's about choosing foods that heal, energize, and align with the Creator's design.

Pantry Staples for the Edenic Diet:

Rolled oats, quinoa, lentils, brown rice

Chickpeas, black beans, split peas

Raw nuts and seeds (almonds, chia, flax, sunflower)

Fresh and frozen fruits and vegetables

Dates, raisins, figs for natural sweetening

Herbs, spices, sea salt, lemon juice, apple cider vinegar

Olive wood or glass cooking utensils (ditch the plastic)

Sample Simple Meals:

Breakfast: Overnight oats with cinnamon, chia, and apple

Lunch: Lentil vegetable stew with greens and brown rice

Dinner: Sweet potato quinoa bowl with tahini drizzle

Snack: Hummus with cucumber slices or a handful of dates and walnuts

Each bite becomes an act of worship and obedience—choosing life, one meal at a time.

3. Spiritual Declarations

Healing the mind and emotions begins with replacing lies with truth. These declarations help reset your internal dialogue:

"I am not bound by fear. YHVH has given me peace and purpose."

"My body is not broken—it is healing."

"I release shame and receive grace."

"My identity is not in my failures, but in the One who formed me."

"I nourish my body with love and intention."

"I choose to walk in alignment with truth, not emotion."

Say them aloud daily—especially when lies surface.

4. Prayer Templates

Sometimes words fail us. These prayer templates help anchor you when emotions, fatigue, or overwhelm try to steal your voice.

Morning Prayer for Alignment:
"YHVH, I invite You into every part of my being today

body, mind, and spirit.

Lead my thoughts. Order my steps.

Help me to nourish myself in ways that honor Your design.

Let my home be a resting place for Your Spirit.

Let my choices bring peace, not pressure.

I choose life today—in what I eat, what I say, and what I believe."

Evening Prayer of Release:
"Father, I release today into Your hands.

Forgive me where I've clung to control, fear, or shame.

Thank You for walking with me, even when I felt weak.

I speak peace over my body, mind, and emotions.

I welcome Your rest and receive Your love."

These tools don't just support healing. They cultivate a lifestyle of intentional restoration.

Let your days become a return to Eden, one choice, one meal, one breath, one prayer at a time.

III. Journal Prompts and Action Plans

Healing is not linear. There will be setbacks, resistance, and days when you wonder if anything is changing. That's why journaling is essential. It becomes your mirror, your reminder, your altar, and your accountability partner.

In Eden, Adam and Eve walked with YHVH in the cool of the day. That kind of communion wasn't just spiritual. It was relational and reflective. Journaling helps you return to that practice: walking with the Creator in quiet honesty, receiving truth, and recording growth.

Why Journaling Matters on This Journey

It tracks transformation – You'll see how your thoughts, choices, and patterns shift over time.

It reveals strongholds – Writing uncovers repeated lies or triggers you may not see in daily life.

It becomes prayer – When words flow from the heart, they become sacred dialogue.

It renews perspective – On the hard days, your past entries remind you of how far you've come.

Reflection Prompts (Use daily or as needed)

1. What is one lie I believed today? What truth does YHVH offer in its place?

2. What did I nourish my body with today? How did it make me feel emotionally and physically?

3. When did I feel closest to peace today? What contributed to that?

4. What emotion showed up today that needs attention, not judgment?

5. Where am I still striving instead of surrendering?

6. How did I create a sanctuary in my space today?

7. What am I thankful for, even in the middle of discomfort?

Declaration Templates

After reflection, it's time to speak life into your body, thoughts, and atmosphere.

"Today, I choose peace over pressure. I am not behind—I am returning."

"I am not my symptoms. I am a sacred vessel under healing."

"I release the need for perfection. I embrace process and presence."

"This journey is not too hard. I was made for alignment."

"I declare that my home is a sanctuary. My body is a temple. My spirit is alive."

Action Planning: From Insight to Implementation

Insight without action leads to spiritual constipation—clogged with truth but stuck in place. Edenic living is about doing something with what you've learned.

Each week, reflect and act:

1. One belief I need to replace this week:

2. One food or product I'm eliminating or replacing:

3. One rhythm or ritual I'm implementing or refining:

4. One space in my home I'm dedicating to peace:

5. One conversation I need to have (with myself, YHVH, or someone else):

Don't try to change everything at once. Choose one Edenic action each week and follow through. Small faithfulness creates lasting transformation.

Encouragement for the Hard Days

There will be days when your skin flares, your emotions rage, or your energy disappears. That does not mean you're failing. It means you're healing in layers.

Write these reminders into your journal on the days when doubt creeps in.

"Healing is happening even when I can't feel it."

"My worth is not measured by my productivity."

"YHVH walks with me in the wilderness, not just the garden."

"I have not gone back to the beginning—I'm walking forward through resistance."

"Rest is not quitting. It's trusting."

IV. Commissioning and Invitation

You're approaching the end of the book, but not the end of the journey. This is a threshold moment—a crossing from reading into becoming, from learning into living.

You were never just meant to survive in the wilderness of modern life. You were made to reclaim Eden—to walk in wholeness, intimacy, and purpose as you were designed from the beginning.

Eden is not just a story in Genesis.

Eden is not just a longing buried in your soul.

Eden is a mission.

A Call to Keep Walking

You are now commissioned to become a keeper of sacred rhythm. A nourisher of truth. A restorer of the breach. A reminder to the world that healing is possible—not because of trends, but because of the timeless design of the Creator.

Your commission is to:

Honor your body as a vessel of divine breath

Align your home as a sanctuary of peace

Renew your mind with truth over lies

Steward your emotions with compassion and boundaries

Feed your spirit with worship, rest, and communion

Walk daily in rhythms that reflect the garden

Eden Was Never Meant to Stay Lost

The world around you is sick, anxious, inflamed, and distracted. But you carry a seed of wholeness, of clarity, of Eden.

This restoration is not just for you. It is for your children, your community, your generation.

Just as Adam and Eve were told to tend and keep the garden, you, too, are called to cultivate spaces of healing and holiness, starting with your own body and home.

You are not leaving Eden behind.

You are becoming an ambassador of it.

An Invitation Forward

So here is your invitation, dear reader and fellow sojourner:

Keep walking in rhythm with your Creator.

Keep choosing nourishment over numbness.

Keep building homes that heal.

Keep speaking words that restore.

Keep resting like healing is holy.

Keep becoming who you were before the world told you otherwise.

Because Eden is not a destination. It is a way of being.

And you—formed from the dust, filled with the breath of Elohim—were born for it.

Welcome back to the garden.

Now, go and walk it out.

20—Why Not Here? Why Not Now?

The Prophets' Vision of Eden and the Call to Us Today

The journey of Eden is not one of nostalgia. It is a mission.

We weren't left with a memory of perfection just to mourn it.

We were handed a blueprint for restoration.

The ache we feel for Eden isn't just grief. It's a holy summons! A sacred longing that pulls us forward into alignment with the design of the Creator. A design that was never revoked. A garden that was never truly abandoned. A promise still waiting to bloom.

I. The Prophets' Vision of Restoration

Scripture does not end in exile. It ends in return.

The prophets looked ahead and saw a time when deserts would bloom, tears would dry, and the land would become like Eden again. Their visions weren't myths or metaphors. They were roadmaps. They saw what YHVH always intended: restoration that touches every part of life—body, land, spirit, and people.

Isaiah 51:3 – "For Jehovah hath comforted Zion; he hath comforted all her waste places, and hath made her wilderness like Eden, and her desert like the garden of Jehovah; joy and gladness shall be found therein, thanksgiving, and the voice of melody."

Ezekiel 36:35 – "And they shall say, This land that was desolate is become like the garden of Eden; and the waste and desolate and ruined cities are fortified and inhabited."

Joel 2:25–26 – "²⁵ And I will restore to you the years that the locust hath eaten, the canker-worm, and the caterpillar, and the palmer-worm, my great army which I sent among you. ²⁶ And ye shall eat in plenty and be satisfied, and shall praise the name of Jehovah your God, that hath dealt wondrously with you; and my people shall never be put to shame."

Isaiah 58:11 – "and Jehovah will guide thee continually, and satisfy thy soul in dry places, and make strong thy bones; and thou shalt be like a watered garden, and like a spring of water, whose waters fail not."

Revelation 22:1–2 – "¹ And he showed me a river of water of life, bright as crystal, proceeding out of the throne of God and of the Lamb, ² in the midst of the street thereof. And on this side of the river and on that was the tree of life, bearing twelve *manner of* fruits, yielding its fruit every month: and the leaves of the tree were for the healing of the nations."

Jeremiah 6:16 – "Thus saith Jehovah, Stand ye in the ways and see, and ask for the old paths, where is the good way; and walk therein, and ye shall find rest for your souls: but they said, We will not walk *therein*."

These were not just theological hopes—they are echoes from Eden.

The prophets called people to turn around and return to the original way. A path that leads not back in time, but forward into fulfillment. Eden isn't a relic of the past. It's the destiny of the faithful.

II. Eden Isn't a Distant Future—It's a Present Invitation

These scriptures are more than poetic promises for the end of days.

They're invitations to participate now.

Eden is not just coming—it's already emerging wherever we align with the Creator's ways.

Every time you choose

> Peace over chaos,
>
> Plants over poison,
>
> Rest over hustle,
>
> Grace over guilt,
>
> Connection over consumption,

You are tending Eden.

Eden is not "out there." It begins within.

You were designed to be a caretaker of wholeness. To partner with the

Creator in the restoration of all things, not just at the end of the age, but at the start of every day.

"Eden was never fully lost—it just needs tending again."

So, ask yourself:

Why not now?

Why not here?

Why not your body, your family, your home, your habits?

Why not this generation?

III. You Are the Proof Eden Still Matters

You are not waiting for someone else to fix what's broken.

You are the one YHVH called to tend, guard, and plant Eden again, right where you are.

Your healing journey is not a side project.

It is a living testimony.

Every meal you make, every rest you honor, every belief you rewrite,

236

every toxin you remove, every prayer you breathe—these are Eden seeds. They matter more than you know.

You are the garden.

You are the caretaker.

You are the proof that Eden is rising again.

Let your life declare:

"As for me and my house, we will return to the garden."

So, what now?

Keep walking.

Keep tending.

Keep choosing alignment over abandonment.

You don't need to wait for perfection. Eden begins where obedience takes root.

In your kitchen.

In your quiet time.

In your breath, your table, your rest, your words.

Don't just long for the garden.

Live it.

Let Eden be restored in your body, your home, your generation.

And let the world look at your life and ask:

"Where did this peace come from?"

And may your answer be:

"From the ancient path. From the garden.

From the Creator who still walks with us in the cool of the day."

Why not here?

Why not now?

Return to the garden.

Renew the design.

Reclaim the whole.

Final Prayer: a blessing for the reader

Beloved one,

May YHVH, the Creator of Heaven and Earth,

breathe fresh life into every part of you—

your body, mind, emotions, and spirit.

May the ache you've carried for wholeness be answered

with the gentle rhythm of Eden restored

in your meals, in your thoughts, in your relationships, and in your rest.

May every stronghold that held you be broken.

May every lie be replaced with truth.

May every root of trauma be pulled up

and planted with peace, hope, and joy.

I bless your home to become a sanctuary of healing.

I bless your table to nourish others as it nourishes you.

I bless your hands to serve.

I bless your voice to declare.

I bless your heart to remain soft before YHVH.

And as you walk out this restoration,

may you never forget:

You were made for Eden.

And Eden was made for you.

Let Eden begin again through you.

In the Name of the One who walked with us in the cool of the day,

and who still calls us back to the garden,

Amen.

References

Bartel, L. R. (2013). Auditory neuroscience and music: Listening, learning, and memory. *Frontiers in Psychology*, 4, 311. doi:10.3389/fpsyg.2013.00311

Belkaid, Y. &. (2017). Homeostatic immunity and the microbiota. *Immunity*, 46(4), 562-576. doi:10.1016/j.immuni.2017.04.008

Berger, R. &. (2010). Healing environment and expressive modalities: A model for intervention with children exposed to disaster. *Journal of Loss and Trauma*, 15(6), 572–593. doi:10.1080/15325024.2010.508874

Bratman, G. N. (2015). The impacts of nature experience on human cognitive function and mental health. *Annals of the New York Academy of Sciences*, 1249(1), 118–136. doi:10.1111/nyas.12740

Buzzell, L. &. (2009). *Ecopsychology: Restoring the Earth, Healing the Mind.* Sierra Club Books.

Cajochen, C. (2007). Alerting effects of light. *Sleep Medicine Reviews*, 11(6), 453–464. doi:10.1016/j.smrv.2007.07.009

Chevalier, G. S. (2012). Earthing: Health implications of reconnecting the human body to the Earth's surface electrons. *Journal of Environmental and Public Health*, 2012, Article ID 291541. doi:10.1155/2012/291541

Cole, S. W. (2015). *Myeloid differentiation architecture of leukocyte transcriptome dynamics in perceived social isolation.* Proceedings of the National Academy of Sciences.

Creswell, J. D. (2005). Affirmation of personal values buffers neuroendocrine and psychological stress responses. *Psychological Science*, 16(11), 846–851. doi:10.1111/j

Cryan, J. F. (2019). The gut microbiome in neurological disorders. *The Lancet Neurology*, 18(2), 136-148. doi:10.1016/S1474-4422(18)30313-5

Fine, A. H. (2015). *Handbook on Animal-Assisted Therapy: Foundations and Guidelines for Animal-Assisted Interventions (4th ed.).* . Academic Press.

Frey, W. H. (1985). *Crying: The Mystery of Tears*. Winston Press.

Jordan, M. &. (2016). *Ecotherapy: Theory, research and practice*. Macmillan International Higher Education.

Kuo, F. E. (2004). A potential natural treatment for attention-deficit/hyperactivity disorder: Evidence from a national study. *American Journal of Public Health*, 94(9), 1580–1586. doi:10.2105/ajph.94.9.1580

Liu, Y. W. (2016). Prevalence of healthy sleep duration among adults-- United States, 2014. *Morbidity and Mortality Weekly Report*, 65(6), 137-141. doi:10.15585/mmwr.mm6506a1

Lowry, C. A. (2007). Identification of an immune-responsive mesolimbocortical serotonergic system: Potential role in regulation of emotional behavior. *Neuroscience*, 146(2), 756–772. doi:10.1016/j.neuroscience.2007.01.067

Mayer, E. A. (2015). Gut/Brain axis and the microbiota. *Journal of Clinical Investigation*, 125(3), 926-938. doi:10.1172/JCI76304

Park, B. J. (2010). The physiological effects of Shinrin-yoku (taking in the forest atmosphere or forest bathing): Evidence from field experiments in 24 forests across Japan. *Environmental Health and Preventive Medicine*, 15(1), 18–26. doi:10.1007/s12199-009-0086-9

Pierce, H. (2011). Negative air ions and their effects on human health and performance. *International Journal of Molecular Sciences*, 12(8), 5516–5534. doi:10.3390/ijms12085516

Popkin, B. M. (2010). Water, hydration, and health. *Nutrition Reviews*, 68(8), 439–458. doi:10.1111/j.1753-4887.2010.00304.x

Porges, S. W. (2011). *The Polyvagal Theory: Neurophysiological Foundations of Emotions, Attachment, Communication, and Self-Regulation*. W. W. Norton & Company.

Porgews, S. W. (2011). *The polyvagal theory: Neurophysiological foundations of emotions, attachment, communication, and self-regulation*. W. W. Norton & Company.

Rohr, R. (2014). *The Naked Now: Learning to See as the Mystics See*. Franciscan Media.

Spiegel K., L. R. (2005). Impact of sleep debt on metabolic and endocrine function. *The Lancet*, 254(9188), 1435-1439. doi:10.1016/S0140-6736(99)01376-8

Stevens, L. J. (2013). Dietary sensitivities and ADHD symptoms: Thirty-five years of research. *Clinical Pediatrics*, 52(6), 537–543. doi:10.1177/0009922813482813

The Holy Bible American Standard Edition. (1901). New York, NY: Thomas Nelson & Sons.

Tilg, H. Z. (2020). The intestinal microbiota fueling metabolic inflammation. *Nature Reviews Immunology*. doi:10.1038/s41577-019-0198-4

U.S. Department of Health and Human Services. (2023). *Our Epidemic of Loneliness and Isolation: The U.S. Surgeon General's Advisory on the Healing Effects of Social Connection and Community*. Retrieved from U.S. Department of Health and Human Services: https://www.hhs.gov/sites/default

Van der Kolk, B. A. (2014). *The body keeps the score: Brain, mind, and body in the healing of trauma.* Viking.

Vingerhoets, A. J. (2016). The riddle of human emotional crying: A challenge for emotion researchers. *Emotion Review*, 8(3), 207–217. doi:10.1177/1754073915586226

Zeki, S. R. (2014). The experience of mathematical beauty and its neural correlates. *Frontiers in Human Neuroscience*, 8, 68. doi:10.3389/fnhum.2014.00068

Zhang, J. W. (2014). An occasion for unselfing: Beautiful nature leads to prosociality. *Journal of Environmental Psychology*, 37, 61–72. doi:10.1016/j.jenvp.2013.11.008

The Eden Way Toolbox

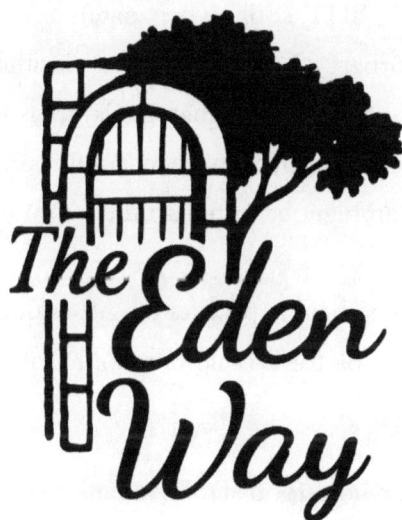

Whole Food Plant-Based Detox Starter Plan

1. Pantry Purge Checklist

☐ Read every label in your pantry, fridge, and freezer.

Ingredient Red Flags: Get Rid of These

☐ High-fructose corn syrup (HFCS)

☐ Monosodium glutamate (MSG)

☐ Artificial sweeteners (aspartame, sucralose, saccharin)

☐ Artificial colors (Red 40, Yellow 5, Blue 1)

☐ Preservatives (BHA, BHT, sodium benzoate)

☐ Emulsifiers (polysorbate 80, carrageenan, soy lecithin)

☐ Hydrogenated or partially hydrogenated oils (trans fats)

☐ Refined seed oils (canola, soybean, corn, sunflower)

☐ "Natural flavors" (ambiguous, often synthetic)

☐ "Artificial flavors"

☐ Aluminum-containing baking powder or anti-caking agents

☐ Synthetic vitamins (look for DL-alpha-tocopherol, cyanocobalamin, etc.)

☐ Replace them with whole-food staples (beans, grains, nuts, fresh produce).

2. Budget Meal Prep

☐ Choose seasonal produce to lower costs and boost nutrients.

☐ Cook a big pot of beans or lentils for the week.

☐ Batch cook whole grains (brown rice, quinoa, barley).

☐ Prepare large Edenic salads with leafy greens, grated veggies, seeds, and oil-free dressing.

☐ Portion leftovers into glass containers or freezer-safe silicone bags.

☐ Keep quick snacks ready: fruit, veggie sticks, hummus, or soaked nuts.

☐ Make one freezer-friendly soup or stew each week.

3. Gentle Healing Tools

☐ Drink 8+ glasses of pure water daily (add lemon or cucumber for extra support).

☐ Start your morning with a warm cup of dandelion or nettle tea.

☐ Add chia seeds or ground flaxseed to smoothies or oatmeal for fiber.

☐ Eat at least 3 servings of non-starchy vegetables daily.

☐ Take time to sweat (gentle exercise or warm bath).

☐ Prioritize restorative sleep (7–9 hours).

☐ Dry brush or gently massage the skin to promote lymphatic drainage.

4. Rebuild with Real Food

☐ Focus on fresh, whole, unprocessed foods—foods without barcodes.

☐ Include fermented foods like sauerkraut, kimchi, or coconut yogurt for gut health.

☐ Eat a rainbow every day (variety of fruits and vegetables).

☐ Incorporate soaked or sprouted nuts and seeds to increase digestibility.

☐ Try green smoothies or blended soups packed with veggies and herbs.

☐ Make 80% of your meals plant-based and oil-free.

☐ Offer gratitude before eating to shift into rest-and-digest mode.

5. Educate Yourself on Whole Food Plant-Based Basics

☐ Learn the difference between vegan and whole food plant-based.

☐ Understand what foods are included: fruits, vegetables, whole grains, legumes, nuts/seeds.

☐ Learn what to avoid: oils, refined flours, added sugars, processed 'plant-based' foods.

☐ Watch a documentary or read a beginner-friendly book (like Forks Over Knives).

☐ Join an online support group or follow WFPB educators for recipes and tips.

6. Stock a WFPB-Friendly Kitchen

☐ Build a core pantry: dry beans, lentils, brown rice, quinoa, oats, amaranth, teff, buckwheat, barley, couscous, corn, whole wheat pasta.

☐ Keep healthy condiments: coconut aminos, balsamic vinegar, tahini, nutritional yeast.

☐ Invest in helpful tools: high-speed blender, Instant Pot, food processor, sharp knives.

☐ Keep frozen fruits and veggies on hand for quick meals and smoothies.

☐ Batch cook simple sauces and dressings to make meals exciting.

7. Keep a Food + Mood Journal

☐ Write down meals and ingredients daily.

☐ Note how you feel 1–2 hours after eating (energy, digestion, mood).

☐ Identify patterns: Do certain foods help you feel clear-headed or bloated?

☐ Track bowel movements, hydration, and emotional cravings.

☐ Reflect on wins each week, no matter how small.

8. Focus on Simple, Repeatable Meals

☐ Pick 3 breakfasts, 3 lunches, and 3 dinners to rotate each week.

☐ Choose 1 new recipe per week to try and learn.

☐ Embrace bowls and mix-and-match meals: grain + bean + veggie + sauce.

☐ Use theme nights: Taco Tuesday, Soup Sunday, Stir-fry Friday.

☐ Keep meals colorful and flavorful with herbs, spices, and citrus.

9. Prepare for Social and Emotional Challenges

☐ Practice a kind, confident response when people question your new way of eating.

☐ Bring your own dish to social gatherings or eat before you go.

☐ Have go-to meals for travel or dining out (chipotle-style bowls, Asian stir-fries, veggie wraps).

☐ Address emotional eating: Are you truly hungry or feeling stressed, tired, or bored?

☐ Find joy in nourishing your body—don't make it about restriction, but about restoration.

10. Pots and Pans Detox

☐ Ditch nonstick cookware (especially Teflon or anything with PTFE/PFOA).

☐ Avoid aluminum cookware, especially uncoated (linked to neurological concerns).

☐ Replace scratched or chipped ceramic pans—coatings can flake into food.

✅ Better Alternatives:

☐ Stainless steel (tri-ply or clad for even heat).

☐ Enameled cast iron (like Le Creuset or Tramontina).

☐ 100% ceramic cookware (Xtrema or similar, lead-free certified).

☐ Glass baking dishes (Pyrex or Anchor Hocking).

11. Utensils Detox

☐ Remove plastic utensils, especially if melted, stained, or warped.

☐ Say goodbye to scratched Teflon-safe tools—they may contain BPA or other leaching plastics.

✅ Better Alternatives:

☐ Wooden utensils (e.g., bamboo, olive wood).

☐ Stainless steel spatulas, ladles, and whisks.

☐ Silicone tools (heat-resistant, food-grade, BPA-free).

12. Storage Containers Detox

☐ Get rid of plastic containers with recycling codes #3 (phthalates), #6 (styrene), and #7 (BPA/unknowns).

☐ Avoid plastic wrap and plastic baggies for hot, fatty, or acidic foods.

☐ Stop reusing single-use plastic containers (takeout boxes, yogurt tubs, etc.) and Ziploc bags.

☐ Plastic cutting boards

✅ Better Alternatives:

☐ Glass containers with snap-lock lids (mason jars, Pyrex sets).

☐ Stainless steel lunchboxes or stackables (like LunchBots or Bento-style tins).

☐ Silicone food storage bags (Stasher, Lerine, or equivalent—BPA-free and freezer safe).

☐ Beeswax wraps for covering bowls or wrapping sandwiches.

☐ Wooden is best for knives, but if you cut meat use glass.

13. Cleaning Tools Detox

☐ Ditch sponge scrubbers with synthetic antimicrobial coatings.

☐ Stop using dish soap with artificial fragrance, triclosan, or sulfates.

☐ Avoid aluminum foil or plastic-lined parchment for high-heat cooking.

✅ Better Alternatives:

☐ Natural bristle dish brushes or compostable sponges.

☐ Plant-based, fragrance-free dish soaps (like Seventh Generation or Dr. Bronner's).

☐ Unbleached parchment or silicone baking mats.

Eden Home Detox Checklist

Creating Sanctuary, Not Just Space

♦ ♦

Bedroom – Detox for Rest and Renewal

☐ Remove synthetic fragrances (air fresheners, candles, sprays)

☐ Replace harsh overhead lighting with soft, warm-toned bulbs

☐ Eliminate blue light sources 1 hour before bed (TVs, phones, etc.)

☐ Use natural fibers for bedding (organic cotton, linen, wool)

☐ Declutter nightstands and under-bed storage

☐ Diffuse calming essential oils (lavender, chamomile, cedarwood)

☐ Add a grounding item like Scripture art, a journal, or a prayer shawl

☐ Designate the room for rest—not work, screens, or chaos

Living Room – Detox for Peace and Presence

☐ Clear clutter from surfaces, shelves, and floors

☐ Replace toxic air fresheners with essential oil diffusers or simmer pots

☐ Play soft, instrumental, or Scripture-based music

☐ Remove spiritually disruptive media (violent, chaotic, or fear-driven content)

☐ Display life-giving reminders (Scripture, affirmations, natural elements)

☐ Include comfortable, conversation-friendly seating

☐ Store blankets, books, or journals in easy reach for calm evenings

Bathroom (Atmosphere Focus—Beyond Products)

☐ Remove visual clutter from counters

☐ Use a plant or stone element to reintroduce nature

☐ Replace synthetic shower curtains with cloth/natural alternatives

☐ Add calming visual elements (art, natural tones, candles)

☐ Keep one drawer or shelf clear for "reset" simplicity

Laundry & Entryway – Detox for Flow and First Impressions

☐ Use non-toxic cleaners and unscented products

☐ Eliminate plastic hampers or containers; replace with baskets or canvas

☐ Add wool dryer balls with essential oils instead of dryer sheets

☐ Create an intentional entry space with hooks, a mat, and calming décor

☐ Declutter shoes, coats, and bags—each item should have a home

Air & Light – Detox the Atmosphere Itself

☐ Open windows daily for fresh air circulation

☐ Use HEPA air purifiers or houseplants that improve indoor air quality (or both)

☐ Let in natural light and remove heavy, dark curtains

☐ Avoid bright white/blue bulbs in the evening

☐ Use beeswax or soy candles (fragrance-free or essential oil-scented)

Digital Detox Zones

☐ Designate one room or corner as a no-device zone

☐ Turn off unnecessary notifications and alerts

☐ Unplug electronics when not in use to reduce EMFs

☐ Create a Sabbath box to rest digital devices weekly

☐ Replace screen time with reading, art, music, or journaling

Sensory Peace Reset

☐ Choose healing soundscapes: nature sounds, Scripture songs, soft music

☐ Reduce overstimulation by limiting media with fast cuts/loud ads

☐ Scent your home intentionally (citrus in the morning, lavender at night)

☐ Include textures like wool, cotton, wood, and stone for tactile grounding

☐ Simplify visual patterns—too many can overstimulate the brain

Spiritual Atmosphere

☐ Pray over every room—dedicate it to its divine purpose

☐ Verbally invite the Ruach: *"Spirit of the Living God, you are welcome here."*

☐ Remove spiritual clutter (occult décor, fear-based media, unspoken tension)

☐ Add sacred anchors: Scripture, candles, prayer corners, worship art

☐ Speak blessings aloud over the home and those who dwell there

Rhythm & Ritual Detox

☐ Establish a morning rhythm (gratitude, prayer, calm music)

☐ Bless meals—even simple ones—with intention and thanks

☐ Create a calming evening wind-down ritual (candle, book, music)

☐ Set a tone of peace before Shabbat—shift music, lighting, and intention

☐ Anchor your family in weekly rhythms that foster safety and connection

Whole-Home Emotional Reset

☐ Identify and release objects that carry grief, shame, or trauma

☐ Replace with items that hold joyful, sacred, or healing memories

☐ Create one dedicated space for joy—dancing, creativity, laughter

☐ Involve your family in shaping the emotional tone of the home

☐ Speak life and truth daily within the walls: *"This is a house of peace."*

Personal Care Detox Checklist

Ditch toxins. Nourish your body. Choose ingredients you can pronounce.

1. Deodorants

☐ Avoid conventional antiperspirants with:
Aluminum compounds (linked to hormonal disruption and possible neurotoxicity)
Fragrance (a blanket term hiding hundreds of chemicals)
Parabens and phthalates

✅ Better Alternatives:

☐ Mineral-based deodorants (like magnesium or baking soda blends)

☐ Crystal deodorants (alum-based but free of aluminum chlorohydrate)

☐ Natural brands: Native, Schmidt's (baking soda-free version), or Earth Mama

☐ DIY deodorant: coconut oil + arrowroot + baking soda (optional) + essential oils

2. Shampoos & Conditioners

☐ Avoid formulas with:
Sodium lauryl/laureth sulfate (SLS/SLES) – harsh detergents
Parabens – endocrine disruptors
Artificial fragrance and dyes
Polyethylene glycols (PEGs) – linked to contamination concerns

✅ Better Alternatives:

☐ Unscented or essential-oil-scented formulas

☐ Castile soap (like Dr. Bronner's) or herbal shampoo bars

☐ Aloe vera-based shampoos

☐ Brands: Pura d'or, 100% Pure, Acure, Alaffia, or Carina Organics

☐ DIY hair rinses: Apple cider vinegar, rosemary tea, nettle rinse

3. Lotions & Body Creams

☐ Avoid these common toxins:
    Mineral oil or petroleum derivatives
    Fragrance/parfum
    Synthetic colors
    Propylene glycol and PEGs

✅ Better Alternatives:

☐ Plant-based oils (jojoba, sweet almond, coconut, shea butter)

☐ Brands: The Naked Bee, Lavido, Earth Mama, or DIY whipped shea butter

☐ Choose unscented versions or essential oil-infused products

4. Makeup

☐ Avoid cosmetics with:
    Talc (especially if not certified asbestos-free)
    Bismuth oxychloride (irritant)
    Fragrance/parfum
    Formaldehyde-releasing preservatives (DMDM hydantoin, etc.)
    Coal tar dyes and heavy metals (often in lipsticks and eyeliners)

✅ Better Alternatives:

☐ Mineral-based and organic makeup brands

☐ Brands: RMS Beauty, 100% Pure, Ilia, Alima Pure, or Crunchi

☐ Lip balms made from beeswax, cocoa butter, and natural oils

☐ Try going makeup-free once a week to let your skin breathe

5. Perfumes & Colognes

☐ Avoid synthetic fragrance blends, which can include:
   Phthalates (hormone disruptors)
   Benzene derivatives and aldehydes (linked to cancer risk and respiratory irritation)

✅ Better Alternatives:

☐ Essential oil rollers (lavender, frankincense, patchouli, citrus)

☐ Natural botanical perfumes (alcohol-free, essential oil-based)

☐ Brands: Heretic, Pacifica, or DIY blends with jojoba oil and essential oils

6. Body Wash & Soaps

☐ Avoid products with:

Sodium Lauryl Sulfate (SLS) and Sodium Laureth Sulfate (SLES) (skin irritants and potential contaminants like 1,4-dioxane)

Parabens (hormone disruptors)

Synthetic fragrance (often containing phthalates and undisclosed chemicals)

Triclosan (linked to antibiotic resistance and endocrine disruption)

✅ Better Alternatives:

☐ Castile-based or plant-based soaps free of synthetic fragrance

☐ Epsom salt-based body washes with natural essential oils

☐ Brands: Dr. Bronner's Pure-Castile Soap, Dr Teal's Body Wash (Eucalyptus, Lavender, or Coconut Oil lines), or homemade blends with liquid castile soap, aloe vera, and essential oils

7-Day Sample Detox Menu

Day 1

Breakfast: Steel-cut oats with berries, ground flax, and cinnamon

Lunch: Lentil soup with kale, carrots, and turmeric

Snack: Apple slices with homemade tahini dip

Dinner: Roasted root vegetables, quinoa, and lemony chickpeas

Drink: Herbal tea and filtered water throughout the day

Day 2

Breakfast: Chia pudding with almond milk, sliced banana, and a dash of vanilla

Lunch: Quinoa tabbouleh with parsley, cucumber, and lemon

Snack: Celery sticks with sunflower seed butter

Dinner: Baked sweet potato, sautéed greens, and herbed lentils

Drink: Ginger tea and cucumber-infused water

Day 3

Breakfast: Smoothie with spinach, pear, ground flax, and unsweetened plant milk

Lunch: Millet bowl with steamed broccoli, avocado, and tahini drizzle

Snack: Cucumber and radish slices with lemon and sea salt

Dinner: Stir-fried mushrooms, zucchini, and brown rice with garlic-free coconut aminos

Drink: Dandelion root tea and filtered water

Day 4

Breakfast: Buckwheat porridge with chopped apple, cinnamon, and walnuts

Lunch: Chickpea salad lettuce wraps with grated carrot and cucumber

Snack: Sliced orange and a handful of pumpkin seeds

Dinner: Roasted cauliflower steak, mashed rutabaga, and steamed asparagus

Drink: Peppermint tea and lemon water

Day 5

Breakfast: Mashed avocado on sprouted grain toast with hemp hearts

Lunch: Barley and black bean salad with fresh cilantro and lime

Snack: Fresh berries and coconut yogurt

Dinner: Cabbage and mushroom stew over wild rice

Drink: Hibiscus tea and mineral-rich herbal infusion (e.g., nettle + oat straw)

Day 6

Breakfast: Warm quinoa with raisins, almond butter, and cinnamon

Lunch: Steamed vegetable medley with tahini-lemon dressing and red lentils

Snack: Apple with cinnamon and raw sunflower seeds

Dinner: Spaghetti squash with garlic-free basil pesto and sautéed greens

Drink: Rooibos tea and plain filtered water

Day 7

Breakfast: Green smoothie with cucumber, kale, green apple, chia, and lime

Lunch: Brown rice nori rolls with grated veggies and avocado

Snack: Baby carrots and beet hummus

Dinner: Butternut squash soup with a side of millet flatbread and shredded cabbage salad

Drink: Chamomile tea and electrolyte-rich coconut water (unsweetened)

Scriptures Showing Yeshua Opposed the Sacrificial System

This appendix lists key scriptures that support the view that Yeshua (Jesus) was not a blood sacrifice in the traditional priestly sense, but rather a prophet and reformer who challenged the corrupt temple sacrificial system. His death was the result of his confrontation with religious power structures, not a divine requirement for animal blood.

Prophetic Challenge to the Temple System

Matthew 21:12–13 – "[12] And Jesus entered into the temple of God, and cast out all them that sold and bought in the temple, and overthrew the tables of the money-changers, and the seats of them that sold the doves; [13] and he saith unto them, It is written, My house shall be called a house of prayer: but ye make it a den of robbers."

This was a direct attack on the sacrificial marketplace inside the temple. The money changers and animal sellers were part of the temple economy. This act threatened the system.

Mark 11:15–18 – "[15] And they come to Jerusalem: and he entered into the temple, and began to cast out them that sold and them that bought in the temple, and overthrew the tables of the money-changers, and the seats of them that sold the doves; [16] and he would not suffer that any man should carry a vessel through the temple. [17] And he taught, and said unto them, Is it not written, My house shall be called a house of prayer for all the nations? but ye have made it a den of robbers. [18] And the chief priests and the scribes heard it, and sought how they might destroy him: for they feared him, for all the multitude was astonished at his teaching."

The decision to kill Yeshua came immediately after he disrupted the temple sacrifices. His act of cleansing the temple was the tipping point.

John 2:14–16 – "¹⁴ And he found in the temple those that sold oxen and sheep and doves, and the changers of money sitting: ¹⁵ and he made a scourge of cords, and cast all out of the temple, both the sheep and the oxen; and he poured out the changers' money, and overthrew their tables; ¹⁶ and to them that sold the doves he said, Take these things hence; make not my Father's house a house of merchandise."

Yeshua physically removed the elements of animal sacrifice, revealing his rejection of the temple's corruption.

Prophecies Against Sacrifice Quoted or Lived by Yeshua

Matthew 9:13 (cf. Hosea 6:6) – "But go ye and learn what *this* meaneth, 'I desire mercy, and not sacrifice'..."

Yeshua quotes Hosea, signaling a shift away from ritual offerings to ethical living.

Matthew 12:7 – "⁷ But if ye had known what this meaneth, I desire mercy, and not sacrifice, ye would not have condemned the guiltless. "

Yeshua connects the rejection of sacrifice with unjust condemnation of the innocent animals—exposing how religious leaders misuse the system.

Temple and Sacrifice as Obsolete

Matthew 24:1–2 – "And Jesus went out from the temple, and was going on his way; and his disciples came to him to show him the buildings of the temple. ² But he answered and said unto them, See ye not all these things? verily I say unto you, There shall not be left here one stone upon another, that shall not be thrown down."

Yeshua prophesies the destruction of the temple, the center of animal sacrifices. He foresaw and likely welcomed its end.

John 4:21–24 – "²¹ Jesus saith unto her, Woman, believe me, the hour cometh, when neither in this mountain, nor in Jerusalem, shall ye worship the Father. ²² Ye worship that which ye know not: we worship that which we know; for salvation is from the Jews. ²³ But the hour cometh, and now is, when the true worshippers shall worship the Father in spirit and truth: for such doth the Father seek to be his worshippers. ²⁴ God is a Spirit: and they that worship him must worship in spirit and truth."

Yeshua shifts worship away from temple ritual—including sacrifice—toward inner transformation and relationship.

Hebrews 10:5–9 (cf. Psalm 40:6–8) – "⁵ Wherefore when he cometh into the world, he saith, 'Sacrifice and offering thou wouldest not, But a body didst thou prepare for me;
⁶ In whole burnt offerings and *sacrifices* for sin thou hadst no pleasure:
⁷ Then said I, Lo, I am come (In the roll of the book it is written of me) To do thy will, O God.' ⁸ Saying above, Sacrifices and offerings and whole burnt offerings and *sacrifices* for sin thou wouldest not, neither hadst pleasure therein (the which are offered according to the law), ⁹ then hath he said, Lo, I am come to do thy will. He taketh away the first, that he may establish the second."

This shows the early believers understood Yeshua's mission as replacing the old system—not continuing it.

The Plot to Kill Him Was Religious, Not Just Political

John 11:47–53 – "⁴⁷ The chief priests therefore and the Pharisees gathered a council, and said, What do we? for this man doeth many signs. ⁴⁸ If we let him thus alone, all men will believe on him: and the Romans will come and take away both our place and our nation. ⁴⁹ But a certain one of them, Caiaphas, being high priest that year, said unto them, Ye know nothing at all, ⁵⁰ nor do ye take account that it is expedient for you that one man should die for the people, and that the whole nation perish not. ⁵¹ Now this he said not of himself: but being high priest that year, he prophesied that Jesus should die for the nation; ⁵² and not for the nation only, but that he might also gather together into one the children of God that are scattered abroad. ⁵³ So from that day forth they took counsel that they might put him to death."

The temple leaders feared losing control, not just to Rome, but over the religious system—including sacrifices.

Acts 6:13–14 (Stephen's trial) – "¹³ and set up false witnesses, who said, This man ceaseth not to speak words against this holy place, and the law: ¹⁴ for we have heard him say, that this Jesus of Nazareth shall destroy this place, and shall change the customs which Moses delivered unto us."

Early followers were accused of attacking the temple system, clearly understood as a central conflict.

Shabbat Read Along

"Shabbat Is Here!"

Shabbat is here, the candles glow,
A quiet peace begins to grow.
The table's set, the bread is warm,
We leave behind the busy swarm.

No school, no chores, no buzzing phone,
It's time to rest, to just be home.
We sing, we pray, we laugh, we eat,
With songs and stories, rest feels sweet.

We light the candles, close our eyes,
And thank the One who made the skies.
The stars peek out to say, "Shalom!"
It's time to let our worries roam.

We build a fort, we take a walk,
We slow things down, we sit and talk.
We draw and read and nap a bit,
And think of heaven—just a split.

For one whole day, we step aside,
And let our hearts in Him abide.
He made the world, then took a break,
And told us all to do the same.

So, every week, from dusk to light,
We welcome peace each Friday night.
Shabbat is more than just a day—
It's love. It's joy. It's Heaven's way.

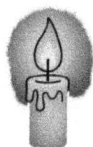

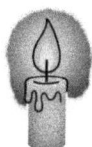

Write Your Own Psalm Below

You can follow the structure—or let it flow however your heart needs.

O YHVH, my _____,

(Write your grief here.)

I cry out to You because_____

_____

_____

_____

(Describe your need.)

Help me, because I feel_____

_____

_____

_____

But I remember_____

_____

_____

_____

(Speak a truth about Him.)

I will choose to trust You because_____

_____

_____

_____

(Make your declaration.)

Blessed be Your Name, even in this. _____

_____

_____

_____

Edenic Living Budgeting Worksheet

This worksheet is designed to help you steward your finances while pursuing Edenic wellness. It's intentionally simple—because managing your money shouldn't be complicated. There is beauty in simplicity, and peace in living within your means.

As you reduce unnecessary spending and align your resources with your values, you'll likely notice less financial stress, more clarity, and greater freedom to invest in what truly matters—your health, your home, and your spiritual life.

How to Use This Worksheet

Begin with Awareness – Take an honest look at your current spending. Where is your money going each month? What categories feel aligned—and which feel excessive or out of balance?

Set Edenic Intentions – Use the space provided to name areas where you can simplify, reduce, or redirect spending. Think through what you truly need versus what is simply habitual or emotionally driven.

Prioritize What Nourishes – Identify one area worth investing in that supports your Edenic wellness—like whole food, movement, healing tools, or rest.

Practice Release – Choose at least one non-essential expense to release this month. Letting go is an act of trust and freedom.

Reflect and Reset Monthly – Return to this worksheet regularly. Stewardship is not about restriction—it's about realignment and ongoing faithfulness.

Use this tool to reflect honestly, spend wisely, and live with joyful intention. The more you simplify, the more space you make for peace.

Monthly Income

Source of Income	Amount
Primary Job	$
Secondary Job	$
Other (e.g., child support, benefits)	$
Total Monthly Income	$

Monthly Expenses

Category	Budgeted	Actual	Difference
Housing (rent/mortgage)	$	$	$
Utilities (electric, water, etc.)	$	$	$
Phone/Internet/Cable/Entertainment	$	$	$
Transportation	$	$	$
Groceries (whole foods)	$	$	$
Wellness (supplements, natural remedies)	$	$	$
Medications	$	$	$
Giving (tithes, donations)	$	$	$
Other	$	$	$
Savings	$	$	$
Investment	$	$	$
Total Expenses	$	$	$

Simplicity and Stewardship Reflection

What is one area I can simplify this month—either in spending, time, or mental clutter?

What is one area worth investing in for my Edenic health— physically, emotionally, or spiritually?

What is one non-essential item, habit, or expense I can release to make space for what matters?

Where have I been spending out of emotion, pressure, or distraction instead of purpose?

How can I invite more beauty and peace into my financial life through simplicity?

What does "enough" look like for me in this season?

How can I practice gratitude with what I already have?

What is one financial habit I want to shift this month toward intentional stewardship?

Final Notes

Edenic stewardship isn't about spending more—it's about aligning your resources with what you value most. It's not about lack—it's about clarity, peace, and purpose. Trust that the Creator multiplies faithfulness, not excess.

Steward with intention.

Walk in peace.

ABOUT THE AUTHOR

Angel Tate Keaton is a writer, teacher, and founder of **Healthy in Heart Media, LLC**, whose journey through chronic illness, emotional trauma, and spiritual burnout led her to a path of healing rooted in the Creator's original design. Blending a background in psychology with deep faith and lived experience, she equips others to reclaim wholeness—body, mind, and spirit.

She is the author of *The Eden Way: Reclaiming Body, Mind, and Spirit* and the creator of *The Eden Way Journal: 49 Days to Reset Body, Mind, and Spirit*, *The Eden Way Workbook*, and its companion, *Nurturing the Journey: The Eden Way Facilitator's Edition*. She continues to expand *The Eden Way* series with upcoming titles and resources.

Angel also leads **RISE with Momentum Circle**, a weekly support group focused on plant-based living, emotional healing, and spiritual renewal.

Born in the quiet hills of Pearisburg, Virginia, she now lives in Roanoke with her husband Todd, their daughter Kelsey, and a handful of quirky cats—plus a few curious "Sabbath-loving ants."

"And thine ears shall hear a word behind thee, saying, 'This is the way, walk ye in it'…" —Isaiah 30:21

⸜ Connect at https://healthyinheart.com and follow on social media @healthyinheart

www.ingramcontent.com/pod-product-compliance
Lightning Source LLC
Chambersburg PA
CBHW022045020426
42335CB00012B/559